Lourdes M. Cuéllar

Diane B. Ginsburg

Preceptor's Handbook for Pharmacists

American Society of Health-System Pharmacists®

Bethesda, MD

Any correspondence regarding this publication should be sent to the publisher, American Society of Health-System Pharmacists, 7272 Wisconsin Avenue, Bethesda, MD 20814, attn: Special Publishing. Produced in conjunction with the ASHP Publications Production Center.

The information presented herein reflects the opinions of the contributors and reviewers. It should not be interpreted as an official policy of ASHP or as an endorsement of any product.

Because of ongoing research and improvements in technology, the information and its applications contained in this text are constantly evolving and are subject to the professional judgment and interpretation of the practitioner due to the uniqueness of each pharmacist's role in precepting students. The editors, contributors, and ASHP have made reasonable efforts to ensure the accuracy and appropriateness of the information presented in this document. However, any reader of this information is advised that the editors, contributors, and ASHP are not responsible for the continued currency of the information, for any errors or omissions, and/or for any consequences arising from the use of the information in the document in any and all practice settings. Any reader of this document is cautioned that ASHP makes no representation, guarantee, or warranty, express or implied, as to the accuracy and appropriateness of the information contained in this document and will bear no responsibility or liability for the results or consequences of its use.

Director of Special Publishing and Acquisitions: Cynthia Conner
Editorial Project Manager: Dana A. Battaglia
Project Editor: Kristin Eckles
Cover and Page Design: Armen Kojoyian

ISBN: 1-58528-116-6

To all who have the passion to teach and to understand the importance of giving back and especially to those who instilled this in us.

Lourdes M. Cuéllar dedicates this book in loving memory of her late parents, Celso and Matiana Cuéllar, and to her siblings, Celso Cuéllar, Jr. and Nicanora (Nicki) C. Cuéllar.

Diane B. Ginsburg dedicates this book in loving memory of her late mother, Phyllis B. Ginsburg.

Table of Contents

Appendix

Acknowledgments

Webster defines *passion* as, "extreme, compelling emotion; intense emotional drive or excitement." When one decides to teach another, it is this emotion, this excitement about seeing others develop that overcomes and satisfies this passion and encourages us to do more. To teach is to have the passion and dedication in others, a true selfless act knowing that others will be the beneficiaries of your time and commitment.

We were very fortunate to have worked with so many others who understand this passion in the writing of this handbook. Certainly anyone who has ever precepted a student knows the importance of giving back to the profession by assisting in the development of its future practitioners. We are grateful to all who have contributed to this work and thank you for your commitment to the future of this profession. We hope this text will be a valuable guide for those who are embarking on this aspect of their practice. There are few things more rewarding than knowing and seeing that you have indeed helped develop another.

We want to thank those who have impressed upon us the importance of giving back, the many students we have taught over the years. All of you have taught us many important lessons and are the reason why we both actively teach today. All of you have touched our lives in immeasurable ways, and we are committed to those who will be teaching in the future.

We want to thank our editors and staff at ASHP for their assistance with the publication of the handbook. We are greatly appreciative of your insight and understanding of the need for this type of guide for practitioners.

In addition, we want to thank the true inspirations in our lives, our late parents, who instilled in each of us the importance of giving back and helping others. We were fortunate to have had such incredible role models in our lives. We honor their memory by our giving to others.

Lourdes M. Cuéllar, MS, R.Ph., FASHP, Editor

Diane B. Ginsburg, MS, R.Ph., FASHP, Editor

Foreword

Who of us does not recall the impact that a parent, sibling, extended family member, friend, or neighbor has had on our life? Whether teaching us our manners around the dinner table or encouraging us to aspire to high expectations, special people affect our lives. These people are oftentimes referred to as mentors. Mentors come in all kinds of styles and patterns. Some are very directive while others let their own lives and works rub off on admirers.

The notion that we all stand on the shoulders of those who have come before us is an appropriate reflection of the meaning of mentors and mentorship. In our personal lives, we are who we are based on our patterning or following in the lead of mentors. Our professional lives have been constructively guided by teachers, administrators, pharmacist preceptors, professional associations, and other role models with whom we have come in contact.

It is from them that we have learned the values and norms of our society, culture, and profession. We learned what is right and wrong, and we came to develop our passions for the care of another human being in our professional roles. They taught us how to relate to other health professionals, and they modeled options for getting out of tough situations.

Mentorship in pharmacy has been a critical element of professional education, training, and development in pharmacy since the advent of the occupation of pharmacy.[1] Passing on the profession's values and ideals to newcomers in the field has been an important element of formal and informal education. This professional socialization plays such a fundamental role in the development of professionals that a philosophical and research literature exists around the issue.[2,3] Moreover, it is a contemporary topic in educational, professional, and policy circles as the nature of health care, the pharmacist's role in the health care system, and the progression of science continues to evolve.[4,5]

Fundamentally, how aspirants in pharmacy immerse themselves into the profession can not be an afterthought in the educational process. Nor can it take a back seat when the degree in pharmacy has been achieved. Adapting to and intrinsically adhering to the norms, values, behaviors, and aspirations of the pharmacy profession is a lifelong behavioral dynamic that affects us all.

Structured pharmacy education in the United States began by incorporating the important aspects of apprenticeship; the modeling of skills and attitudes after the master craftsman. The early curricula offered by the founding schools of pharmacy in the first several decades of the 19th century were built on the skills taught by "master pharmacists" during the daytime work in the shops and then augmented by lectures in the evening in which the fledgling science of pharmacy was taught.[6] Dr. Albert Prescott of the University of Michigan challenged that notion and was an early advocate of bringing all teaching into the University setting and leaving "apprenticeship" in pharmacy in the hands of the practice outside of the control and domain of the university.[7] Changes in educational philosophy and practice in the 1960s brought structured experiential education into better balance with didactic instruction in schools and colleges of pharmacy.[8] The contemporary pharmacy curriculum requires an extensive, structured experiential component in order to give student pharmacists practice opportunity in traditional, diverse, and unique practice sites under the supervision of faculty and practitioner preceptors.[9]

In that process, important philosophical precepts of practice are directly and indirectly taught. Even bad experiences in such relationships serve as important educational and developmental lessons.

When thinking about practitioner development, there exist many similarities between a mentoring and precepting relationship. Both focus on the need to establish an effective relationship between the leader and the pupil that fosters growth, offers constructive feedback, and provides a "safe" environment for reflection and assessment.[10] Leadership in these relationships require an effectual role model who is qualified in the subject matter and willing/available to advise and guide his/her pupils.

Differences among precepting and mentoring are based on the goals, structure, and duration of the relationship between leader and pupil.[11] A precepting relationship aims to develop the professional and/or instructional growth of a pupil, usually taking place in a structured environment for a specified time, which enables the pupil to apply theories learned.[12] A mentoring relationship aims to encourage the personal and/or professional growth of a pupil, usually taking place in an unstructured environment with no time frame, which enables the pupil to develop and test theories.

It is very possible for a precepting relationship to evolve into a mentoring relationship. Initially, most precepting relationships tend to be hierarchical, with very clear lines of authority between the leader and the pupil. However, over time those lines can begin to fade. Through a precepting relationship, individuals can be naturally drawn to each other by similar interests, values, or characteristics—providing the opportunity for both leader and pupil to learn from each other and creating more of a mentoring relationship. Therefore, even after a formal precepting relationship has concluded, a bond between the leader and pupil can continue to flourish providing mutual benefits for both.

Cuéllar, Ginsburg, and their colleagues describe the importance of this aspect of practitioner development and of mentorship on the pages that follow. Different perspectives on mentoring and the dynamics of personal and professional socialization are outlined. But most importantly, an understanding of the role that mentoring plays in moving oneself to personal and professional excellence is well-underscored by all of the contributing authors.

In a way, mentoring is a gift that is equally shared by the one providing the mentoring and the person benefiting from the mentor relationship. It is then a process that should be valued and celebrated. This book gives credence to this point: the reader will be better for having read and thought about the mentoring process and its impacts. Further, it is my hope that the readers of this book will strengthen their own commitments to become mentors of excellence to the generations of aspiring pharmacists that follow.

Henri R. Manasse, Jr., Ph.D., Sc.D.
Executive Vice President and Chief Executive Officer
American Society of Health-System Pharmacists
Bethesda, Maryland

September, 2004

References

1. Manasse Jr., HR. Unpublished Ph.D. Dissertation. University of Minnesota; 1974.
2. Friedson E, (ed.). *The Professions and Their Prospects.* Beverly Hills, CA: Sage Publications; 1973.
3. Becker HS, Geer B, Hughs EC, et al. *Boys in White: Student Culture in Medical School.* New Brunswick, NJ: Transaction Publishers; 1991.
4. American Associate of Colleges of Pharmacy. White paper on pharmacy student professionalism. Available at: http://www.aacp.org/Docs/MainNavigation/ForStudentsApplicants/6056_1999WhitePaperProfessionalism.pdf. Accessed September 17, 2004.
5. American Society of Health-System Pharmacists. *Professionalism in Pharmacy.* Unfinished and New Business: Proceedings of the 2004 Annual ASHP House of Delegates Session. ASHP 2004 Summer Meeting: June 20–22, 2004; Las Vegas, NV. Edited by Manasse HR, 2004.
6. Kremers E, Urdang G. *Kremers and Urdang's History of Pharmacy* (revised by Glenn Sonnedecker). Philadelphia, PA: Lippincott; 1963.
7. Manasse Jr., HR. Innovation, confrontation, and perseverance—Albert B. Prescott's legacy to pharmaceutical education in America. *Pharm Hist.* 1973;15(1):22–8.
8. Manasse HR, Nona DA, Betz RP. Experience requirement for pharmacy practice. *J Am Pharm Assoc.* 1972;12(5):210–4.
9. Accreditation Council for Pharmacy Education. Accreditation standards and guidelines for the professional program in pharmacy leading to the doctor of pharmacy degree. Available at: http://www.acpe-accredit.org/standards/standards1.asp#3. Accessed September 17, 2004.
10. Preceptor & Mentor Initiative for Health Sciences in BC. Role similarities. Available at: www.bcahc.ca/pm/managingprograms/precepting-vs-mentoring/role-similarities.htm. Accessed August 12, 2004.
11. Ibid. Role differences. Available at: www.bcahc.ca/pm/managingprograms/precepting-vs-mentoring/role-differences.htm. Accessed August 12, 2004.
12. Trovato J, Edwards J. Education and training of pharmacy students. *Am J Health-Syst Pharm.* 2004;61:1956–7.

Editors

Lourdes M. Cuéllar, MS, R.Ph., FASHP
Sr. Executive Director
Medical Support Services
Director of Pharmacy
The Institute for Rehabilitation and Research (TIRR)
Houston, Texas

Diane B. Ginsburg, MS, R.Ph., FASHP
Clinical Associate Professor
Assistant Dean for Student Affairs
College of Pharmacy
The University of Texas at Austin
Austin, Texas

Contributors

Linda Stevens Albrecht, MBA, R.Ph., FASHP
Clerkship Coordinator
College of Pharmacy
The University of Texas at Austin
Dallas/Fort Worth Region, Texas

Randy Ball, MBA, R.Ph.
Director of Pharmacy
Harris Methodist Fort Worth Hospital
Fort Worth, Texas

Lourdes M. Cuéllar, MS, R.Ph., FASHP
Sr. Executive Director
Medical Support Services
Director of Pharmacy
The Institute for Rehabilitation and Research (TIRR)
Houston, Texas

Nicanora C. Cuéllar, MSW, LCSW, DCSW, C-ASWCM, C-SWHC
Senior Social Worker
Pediatric Rheumatology Center
Texas Children's Hospital
Houston, Texas

Debra S. Devereaux, MBA, R.Ph., FASHP
DUR Manager
School of Pharmacy
University of Wyoming
Laramie, Wyoming

Steven H. Dzierba, R.Ph., MS, FASHP
Associate Team Manager
Clinical Education
Pfizer Incorporated
Southlake, Texas

Frederick M. Eckel, MS, R.Ph.
Professor
School of Pharmacy
University of North Carolina
Executive Director
North Carolina Association of Pharmacists
Chapel Hill, North Carolina

Dana S. Fitzsimmons, R.Ph., MBA, FASHP
Associate Team Manager
Clinical Education
Pfizer, Incorporated
Washington, DC

Diane B. Ginsburg, MS, R.Ph., FASHP
Clinical Associate Professor
Assistant Dean for Student Affairs
College of Pharmacy
The University of Texas at Austin
Austin, Texas

Christine E. Huls, R.Ph., Pharm.D.
Pharmacist, Clinical Specialist
Department of Pharmacy
The Institute for Rehabilitation and Research (TIRR)
Houston, Texas

Grace M. Kuo, R.Ph., Pharm.D.
Assistant Professor of Family and Community Medicine
Baylor College of Medicine
Houston, Texas

Sarah Lake-Wallace, Pharm.D., R.Ph.
Pharmacy Administrator of Clinical Services
Pharmacy Department
Kelsey-Seybold Clinic
Houston, Texas

David Lorms, CAE
Director
Association Management Development and Regional Liaison
Member and Affiliate Relations and Forums
American Society of Health-System Pharmacists
Bethesda, Maryland

Darlene M. Mednick, R.Ph., MBA, NPDP, PAHM, FAMCP
Senior Vice President and COO
Chief Pharmacy Officer
Navitus Health Solutions, LLC
Madison, Wisconsin

Traci L. Metting, R.Ph., Pharm.D.
Director
Clinical Pharmacy
Broadlane, Incorporated
Dallas, Texas

John E. Murphy, Pharm.D.
Department Head
Pharmacy Practice and Science
Assistant Dean
College of Pharmacy
University of Arizona
Tucson, Arizona

Jennifer R. Myhra, R.Ph.
Clinical Associate Professor
Assistant Dean for Experiential and Professional Affairs
College of Pharmacy
University of Texas at Austin
Austin, Texas

Ruth E. Nemire, BSPh., Pharm.D., R.Ph.
Director
Office of Community Outreach
Assistant Professor
Department of Pharmacy Practice
College of Pharmacy
Health Professions Division
Nova Southeastern University
Fort Lauderdale, Florida

Michael Piñón, R.Ph., Pharm.D.
Clinical Coordinator
Sierra Medical Center
El Paso, Texas
Clinical Assistant Professor of Pharmacy Practice
Texas Tech University
El Paso, Texas

Vikki Jill Polk, R.Ph., Pharm.D.
Pharmacy Resident
College of Pharmacy
The University of Texas at Austin
Levelland, Texas

Kevin Purcell, MD, R.Ph., Pharm.D., MHA, FASHP, CHE
Healthcare Leaders 2B/Pediatric Research 4U
Leadership Coach and Clinical Investigator
Clinical Associate Professor of Pediatrics
College of Medicine
Texas A&M University
Corpus Christi, Texas

Rita R. Shane, R.Ph., Pharm.D., FASHP
Director
Pharmacy Services
Cedars-Sinai Medical Center
Los Angeles, California
Assistant Dean
Clinical Pharmacy
School of Pharmacy
University of California at San Francisco
San Francisco, California

Kali S. Sommer, R.Ph., Pharm.D.
Drug Education Coordinator
Kaiser Permanente
San Francisco, California (Practice Site)
New Practitioner Executive Committee
American Society of Health-System Pharmacists
San Francisco, California

Stacy A. Taylor, R.Ph., Pharm.D.
Educational Affairs Chairman
Texas Society of Health-System Pharmacists
Clinical Pharmacist
St. Joseph's Regional Health Center
Bryan, Texas

Lee C. Vermeulen, R.Ph., MS
Director
Center for Drug Policy
University of Wisconsin Hospital and Clinics
Clinical Associate Professor
Madison School of Pharmacy
University of Wisconsin
Madison, Wisconsin

If a teacher is indeed wise he does not bid you enter the house of his wisdom, but rather leads you to the threshold of your own mind.

Kahil Gibran

Preface

As a child I was taught that people appreciate you far more for what you do and how you treat others, rather than for what you say you will do or for any material wealth you may have. How do you measure the worth of the outstanding preceptors and mentors that have come into our lives? Each one of us demonstrates or exemplifies characteristics or skills that we learned along the path toward becoming the pharmacists we are today.

There are many individuals that have contributed toward my development as a pharmacist and as an effective pharmacy manager and leader. While I was still in pharmacy school, my long time friend and colleague, Grace Salazar, and I were the first two women to work in the pharmacy at the VA Hospital in Houston. Back then as today, the VA was responsible for dispensing thousands of prescriptions for inpatients and outpatient veterans in our community on a daily basis. The pharmacists at the Houston VA taught me how to respond in a highly stressful environment, how to focus on one patient at a time regardless of the workload, how to communicate with empathy and understanding, and how to be part of a team. They set the bar high, guided me through the learning process, and always provided positive feedback.

From my brother, Celso Cuéllar, who is a long time community pharmacist, I learned how to talk to patients at a level they can understand in a respectful and culturally appropriate manner, how pharmacists can truly become extended members of many of their patients' families, and how empathy, kindness and good listening skills are often the best tools toward affecting compliance and effective medication management.

From the physicians, nurses, pharmacists, technicians, administrative support staff, and other colleagues at The Institute for Rehabilitation and Research where I work, I have learned and continue to learn the true meaning of compassion, collaboration, and teamwork. Being an active member and officer of both my local and state health-system pharmacy organizations also gave me the opportunity to grow personally and professionally.

My colleagues and fellow directors of pharmacy in the Texas Medical Center have facilitated my development as an effective pharmacy leader. We have shared experiences, sought advice from one another, and continue to collaborate on issues pertinent to the profession. From my friend, colleague, and coeditor of this book, Diane Ginsburg, I learned the art of networking and the value of becoming involved with professional organizations at the national level. In addition, she has given me numerous opportunities to develop and advance professionally. Her commitment to students and young practitioners as a teacher, counselor, mentor, and friend is truly commendable.

The need for proficient, energetic preceptors has never been greater. This book is designed to provide pharmacists with critical information about preceptor programs around the U.S. and to help preceptors design a dynamic and effective experiential program at their practice site. We tried to identify topics that we felt would be important for preceptors at all levels and sites of practice (hospital, community, industry, faculty, etc.). This book is meant to be comprehensive, and topics and sections are organized by common areas of skills or proficiencies.

To be an effective preceptor, a pharmacist should exhibit clinical competency skills, possess excellent written and verbal communication skills, and also demonstrate humanistic skills such as listening, compassion, empathy, and observation. Diane Ginsburg and I invited pharmacists from around the U.S. that exemplify the characteristics of exemplary preceptors. In addition, authors were invited who had expertise in their respective areas and brought perspective from different parts of the country and different or unique practice programs. The intent is for this book to be reflective on broad practice guidelines.

One of the greatest satisfactions you can have as a pharmacist today is mentoring students and young practitioners. I am still in contact with the very first student I had the privilege to precept. It is hard to express into words the pride and satisfaction one feels as students you have mentored and precepted develop into outstanding professionals and clinicians.

How do you measure the worth of exemplary preceptors and mentors? You cannot. You thank them for their selfless contributions by practicing and enhancing the skills and training they provided to you. Most importantly, you pass these gifts on to the next generation of practitioners.

Lourdes M. Cuéllar
March, 2005

Modeling may not only be the best way to teach, it may be the only way to teach.

Albert Schweitzer

Chapter 1

Origins of Precepting and Mentoring

Kevin Purcell

Objectives

- Explain the theories of precepting and mentoring dating back to Greek times and mythology.
- Describe current concepts of precepting and mentoring.

The theories of precepting and mentoring have existed for a long time and can be traced back to Greek times and mythology. The earliest reference to precepting can be found in the Hippocratic oath written around 400 B.C. by the great Greek physician Hippocrates (Figure 1-1).[1,2] Hippocrates defined a set of very compelling duties and responsibilities of the physician preceptor in his famous oath. A strong and enduring commitment was formed as the art of medicine was passed down from father to son and from preceptor to student.

The word *mentor* comes from *The Odyssey,* written in approximately 700 B.C. by the Greek poet Homer.[3] Mentor was the name of a wise and loyal advisor and friend of Odysseus, the King of Ithaca. When Odysseus set sail with his army on a long voyage to go fight in the Trojan War, he entrusted his entire household and the direction and teaching of his son Telemachus to Mentor. Athena, daughter of Zeus and Goddess of Wisdom, often appeared disguised in the form of Mentor when providing advice to Telemachus. According to mythology, through Mentor's guidance Telemachus matured to manhood and became an effective leader.

Today the concepts of precepting and mentoring are alive and vital to the professional growth and development of pharmacy students and pharmacists and to the future of the pharmacy profession. Precepting can be defined as teaching others the art and science of pharmacy practice in a health care setting (community pharmacy, hospital, clinic, etc.) with the goal of developing competent practitioners. We rely on experienced practitioners to become preceptors and to pass down to their preceptees knowledge and experience. Precepting involves a partnership for education, investment of time and energy, negotiation and individualization of learning activities, teamwork, coaching, evaluation of performance, and professionalism role modeling and guidance (Figure 1-2). Preceptors assure that their preceptees attain competency at the practice of pharmacy much in the same way that master craftsmen supervise apprentices in developing the skills of their trade. Service is exchanged for education and training.

Mentoring can be defined as helping others reach their full potential as professionals with the goal of developing practitioners who will pursue and attain excellence as patient care providers, teachers, scientists, managers, and/or lead-

Figure 1-1 • Hippocratic Oath

I swear by Apollo Physician and Asclepios and Hygeia and Panacea and all the gods and goddesses, making them my witnesses, that I will fulfill according to my ability and judgment this oath and this covenant:

To hold him who has taught me this art as equal to my parents and to live my life in partnership with him, and if he is in need of money to give him a share of mine, and to regard his offspring as equal to my brothers in male lineage and to teach them this art—if they desire to learn it—without fee and covenant; to give a share of precepts and oral instruction and all other learning to my sons and to the sons of him who has instructed me and to the pupils who have signed the covenant and have taken an oath according to the medical law, but to no one else.

I will apply dietetic measures for the benefit of the sick according to my ability and judgment; I will keep them from harm and injustice.

I will neither give a deadly drug to anybody if asked for it, nor will I make a suggestion to this effect. Similarly, I will not give to a woman an abortive remedy. In purity and holiness I will guard my life and my art.

I will not use the knife, not even on sufferers from stone, but will withdraw in favor of such men as are engaged in this work.

Whatever houses I may visit, I will come for the benefit of the sick, remaining free of all intentional injustice, of all mischief, and in particular of sexual relations with both female and male persons, be they free or slaves.

What I may see or hear in the course of treatment or even outside of the treatment in regard to the life of men, which on no account one must spread abroad, I will keep to myself, holding such things shameful to be spoken about.

If I fulfill this oath and do not violate it, may it be granted to me to enjoy life and art, being honored with fame among all men for all time to come; if I transgress it and swear falsely, may the opposite of all this be my lot.

Translated by Ludwig Edelstein

---

ers. Mentoring is a relationship based on the following: trust and respect; education and nurturing; inspiration to advance the practice of pharmacy and improve patient care; opportunities to grow and develop; metamorphosis through

Figure 1-2 • The Elements of Precepting

P	artnership
R	ole modeling
E	ducation
C	oaching
E	valuation
P	rofessionalism
T	eamwork
I	nvestment
N	egotiation
G	uidance

engaging in a process of self-reflection, self-assessment, and self-transformation; professional guidance; and nomination for awards when success has been achieved (Figure 1-3). We depend on preceptors to also become mentors and help their mentees attain professional excellence and become leaders. Pharmacy preceptors and mentors provide the most critical aspects of professional education and training and truly can make a difference in the lives and careers of their preceptees and mentees.

Figure 1-3 • The Elements of Mentoring

M	etamorphosis
E	ducation
N	urturing
T	rust
O	pportunity
R	espect
I	nspiration
N	omination
G	uidance

References

1. Edelstein L. The genuine works of Hippocrates. *Bull Hist Med.* 1939;7:236–8.
2. Edelstein L. The Hippocratic oath: text, translation, and interpretation. *Bull Hist Med.* 1943;(suppl 1).
3. Homer. *The Odyssey.* Translated by Rieu EV. London, England: Penguin Books; 1946.

You cannot hope to build a better world without improving the individuals. To that end each of us must work for his own improvement, and at the same time share a general responsibility for all humanity, our particular duty being to aid those to whom we think we can be most useful.

Marie Curie

Chapter 2

Goals of Experiential Training

Fred M. Eckel, Traci L. Metting, Ruth Nemire

Chapter Outline

The actual is limited, the possible immense.

La Martine

Differentiating Between Cognitive and Affective Learning

Ruth Nemire

Objectives

- Discern nuances of cognitive, behavioral, and affective learning.
- Develop a teaching method that recognizes that all students are not equal when it comes to learning.
- Employ the basics of Bloom's taxonomy when completing assignments.
- Implement a student-centered approach to learning.

Learning Theories for Preceptors and Students

There are theories, taxonomies, ideologies, and studies about the way a person learns. The question here might be, Why discuss methods of learning at the beginning of a chapter on experiential education? Certainly the way a student learns is no concern for the teacher; it is a concern for the student only. Or is it? Educators have learned that it is really the teacher and those in charge of the curricula who should be as concerned with how students learn as with the facts they learn. This idea was responsible for a movement in the last 20 years in medical education to adopt a problem- or outcomes-based approach to teaching. Both of these approaches are ways of helping students to learn and to meet goals and objectives set by faculty. It is easy to argue that experiential education is a problem- or outcomes-based approach to teaching students, but in many settings it is not. It is important to understand the background of how students learn in order to put in place standards at the experiential rotation site that affect the students' learning of knowledge, skills and application, and attitude.

In order to keep this discussion brief, only the cognitive, behavioral, and affective taxonomy developed by Bloom and associates will be discussed. This taxonomy was developed shortly after World War II when veterans were returning home and going to college and there was a need identified to assess whether students were being evaluated appropriately. At the University of Chicago, Professor Bloom, the director of the Examiner's office, developed the taxonomy as a means of assessment. Over time it has become a mantra for educators when discussing a means to learning. It was never meant to be a theory or philosophy, just a means to assess student learning.[1]

It is important for preceptors to learn and employ the basics of this taxonomy, so that appropriate assessment of student learning is made when developing activities and objectives for a course. Cognitive and affective learning both describe an acquisition of knowledge, skills, or attitudes during the course of an individual experience (Table 2.1). The taxonomies have been called lower-order learning, starting with just the facts or knowledge and then moving up the scale to higher order. Students can actually learn in any order and should be encouraged to do so. As the discussion continues of cognitive versus affective learning, keep in mind the original intention; it will guide you in helping to assess what students are learning.[1]

Cognitive learning is the acquisition of knowledge and information followed by the development of concepts relating to course content. The basics of assessing this kind of learning are multiple-choice type questions that seek to find what facts students know or have memorized for the examination. There is no guarantee that at the most basic cognitive functioning level, students can incorporate these facts into anything useful.[1–3] Behavioral learning is seldom discussed, but it should be defined and addressed, especially in the setting of experiential education. It is the acquisition of skills and development of

Table 2.1 • *Taxonomy from Bloom, Krathwohl, and Masia*[6]

Cognitive Learning	Or	Affective Learning	Or
Knowledge	*Has data*	*Receiving*	*Accepts*
Comprehension	*Understands*	*Responding*	*Takes action*
Application	*Treats*	*Valuing*	*Respects*
Analysis	*Investigates*	*Organizing*	*Manages*
Synthesis	*Blends*	*Internalizing*	
Evaluation	*Appraises*		

Source: References 1–3.

competence in performance of procedures, operations, methods, and techniques. In experiential education for pharmacy students, these could be the technical skills of making or dispensing an intravenous admixture. In the area of patient care, developing methods for assessment of patient therapeutic plans, patient histories, and disease state management education are just a few examples of affective learning.[1–3] While there is no published taxonomy for this in the literature, affective learning can be simple motor tasks that must be learned, but to move toward competence in performance of procedures, methods, and techniques requires the integration of cognitive and affective learning.[4]

The hierarchy of affective learning involves the development of attitudes, feelings, and preferences.[1–3] Within this taxonomy of affective learning, the assessment of learning becomes a quagmire. It is difficult to assess receiving, responding, valuing, organizing, and internalizing of information by the learner. Assessment of this kind of learning in students will be through their professional presentation or their ability to organize and relay information to others.

Students can be seen as empty computer disks. It is the job of the teachers to help the students create files on the disk. Each student who enters the training site may learn a little differently. While facts are important, it is the concepts and application of knowledge and desire to learn that will stay with students. In medicine the facts change regularly, and to keep up many preceptors need to modify years of experience using the same goals and objectives.

Student-Centered Learning vs. Teacher-Centered Learning

Teaching and learning often go on separately, despite the teacher's best efforts. A teaching method can be defined as the "vehicle or technique for instructor-student communication."[4] Learning can occur during reading, writing, reflection, both with and without a teacher, in groups, individually, on purpose, and by accident. It is often education that gets in the way of learning. Student- and teacher-centered concepts are exactly that, and learning revolves around either what the teacher believes students should learn or around the students.

Many people in faculty roles today were taught the teacher-centered model of education. In this passive approach to learning, the teacher stands in the front of the classroom and information is brought forth to fill what can be described as empty computer chips in students' heads. When this occurs, students have little time to file the information in a format that is retrievable for later use. Students may hear every word the professor says, and they may even manage to write everything down on paper. Neither of these actions requires that students process the information, and students are passive learners (if at all). The teacher-centered approach has been shown by educational researchers to be best left to history. It is time to adopt a student-centered approach to learning.

The educational reform that moved the focus to the student began in 1997 with the American Psychological Association.[5] In this approach the teacher does not necessarily stand up in front of a class or decide exactly which data students will learn or how it is learned. This requires an active approach on the part of students; when engaged, students will learn (Table 2.2).[1,4,6,7] Under ideal conditions, students will learn if they are actively involved and if what is being learned affects their inner selves. Student have to find the information personally important. In the classroom or even on experiential education courses, students often do not learn what a faculty member thinks they should because students do not sense a need.[1]

In order to promote learning, preceptors must be authentic and accepting of students rather than thoughtless and uncaring. Many colleges or schools of pharmacy require that students send a resumé or curriculum vitae before attendance at a site. These documents help faculty members understand student accomplishments and create an expectation that students have some prior

Table 2.2 • *Comparison of Instructional Styles*

Teacher-Centered Activities	Student-Centered Activities
Passive	*Active*
Rewards students who can memorize well but not transfer data to other applications	*Rewards researchers, questioners, and problem solvers*
Primary responsibility to relay data to a group	*Small group discussions*
Communication, one way (i.e., lecture)	*Group projects*
Questioning	*Reflective activities*
Demonstration	*Peer teaching* *Role playing*

Source: Adapted from references 4 and 8.

learning. It is important to promote what students know and to facilitate their learning based on that. It is important to help students find a new perspective or insight into the information they need to learn. Preceptors must be able to relate to students on some level in order to have an impact on the learning.[9]

These ideal conditions may seem too difficult to achieve in a setting in which the primary responsibility of preceptors is to do their job as opposed to teaching students. There are ways to accomplish both effectively and perhaps improve performance at all levels. A good teacher will learn from his or her students. It is not enough to just engage students in activities and expect them to learn. Learners need support, guidance, and a chance to reflect on what they know and what they need to know. It is not always the responsibility of the preceptor to provide this for students. Students do well when involved in groups with their peers for various reasons. They learn in groups because they have the opportunity to brainstorm, to present ideas, and to have ideas evaluated, rejected or remodeled, and improved. Small groups increase the commitment of each student. Students have changes in attitudes and behaviors when small groups are used. In some cases, cognitive learning may not be affected, but the affective learning most certainly will.[9]

This student-centered approach may initially cause challenges to preceptors. If students have never been exposed to this method, they will not immediately know how to act, may appear not to be learning, and may be defensive in their new role. Writing has often been a common method for learning. When students engage in writing by answering directed questions or in free-flow discussion of a topic, they write what they know and they learn what they do not. Students often initially rebel against free-flow discussion and writing, but many will learn that reflection helps them, and that is the point.

The EXPLORE (examine, pair, listen, organize, research, and evaluate) process has been used by faculty to create constructive learning. Students are first presented with a controversial statement and asked to commit themselves to a position relating to the issue. Pairs are created from two students who are on opposing sides of the controversy. Each person listens to the other's view so he or she can summarize it accurately. Once the sides have been heard, the students put this issue into a compare-and-contrast table. Then they research the issue to find supporting literature about either side. The pair then compare their findings and agree on research-based statements.[10] Employing any or all of these techniques will help students become better learners. The difficulty is often in the reasoning and motivation of the students.

It has been suggested by Pierce that if students do not view an assignment as appropriate, they should be allowed to identify and create an alternative assignment that will meet the same outcomes.[10] This will likely require patience and direction by the preceptor. At the end of the rotation, students should reflect on each assignment and the amount and value of the learning caused by each. If the assignment was not helpful in learning, this should also be stated and supported.[10] The teacher-centered method of teaching is relied on heavily, for the very reason that it may not pose as many difficulties as the learner-centered approach. Teachers who lecture and are only concerned with knowledge may not be put on the spot with questions. They are able to control the direction of lectures and of the classroom. When the learner-centered approach is employed, students should be encouraged to ask questions and topics may change; preceptors must be able to adapt and move with the learning. It may feel as if all control of the topic has been relinquished to the students. If that occurs, then there is where the learning starts.[11]

These few tricky situations may cause a bit of unease at first, not only for preceptors but also for the students as they "learn to learn." In the end, moving in this direction may be unexpected—an adventure in learning.[11] Preceptors must find their level of comfort and ability to adapt to students with multiple learning styles. Numerous studies attempt to identify one kind of teaching method as better than another, but without success. However, that does not mean teachers should ignore the fact that students have reported more enjoyable learning experiences and changes in attitudes with the learner-centered approach.[4] Table 2.3 matches Bloom's domains of learning with methods of instruction that help students attain those levels. Many students make it to their experiential education courses and have not yet learned *how* to learn. It is these students that may pose the most difficulty for preceptors when employing methods that encourage student-centered learning.

It is important for both full-time faculty and the many adjunct professors and preceptors to recognize Bloom's taxonomy when evaluating what students have learned and to develop a method of teaching that recognizes that all

Table 2.3 • *Matching Domain and Level of Learning to Appropriate Methods*

Domain and Level of Learning from Bloom's Taxonomy	Method
Cognitive	
Knowledge	*Lecture, programmed instruction, drill, and practice*
Comprehension	*Lecture, programmed instruction*
Application	*Discussion, simulation and games, field experience, laboratory*
Analysis	*Discussion, independent/group projects, simulations, field experience, role playing, laboratory*
Synthesis	*Independent/group projects, field experience, role playing, laboratory*
Evaluation	*Independent/group projects, field experience, role playing, laboratory*
Affective	
Receiving	*Lecture, discussion, field experience*
Responding	*Discussion, simulations, role playing, field experience*
Valuing	*Discussion, independent/group projects, simulations, role playing, field experience*
Organization	*Discussion, independent/group projects, field experience*

Source: Reference 4.

students are not equal when it comes to learning. Preceptors need to recognize that learning and teaching do not necessarily occur simultaneously, and that it is within their realm of responsibility to facilitate learning. Students need to learn to think like pharmacists, to be problem-solvers, and to become lifelong learners. They must learn to reflect, evaluate, validate, and verify. These skills are not inherent—students must be taught to learn, and that is where the teachers and preceptors of the new millennium must lead.

References

1. Shulman L. Making differences: a table of learning. *Change.* 2002;November/December:36–44.
2. Lopez C. *Opportunities for Improvement: Advice from Consultant-Evaluators on Programs to Assess Student Learning.* Chicago: North Central Association of Colleges and Schools; March 1996 (reprinted April 1997). ERIC Document Reproduction Service No. ED 463 790.
3. Leith, K. Adult learning styles and the college classroom. Paper presented at: Annual Meeting

of the American Psychological Association; August 22–25, 2002; Chicago. EDRS Document Reproduction Service No. ED470 010 CG 032 020.

4. Weston C, Cranton P. Selecting instructional strategies. *J High Educ.* 1986;57:259–83.
5. Dembo H. Don't lose sight of the students. *Princip Leadership.* 2004;4:37–42.
6. Schwartz W. Education in the classroom. *J High Educ.* 1980;51:235–54.
7. Spencer J, Jordan R. Learner centered approaches in medical education. *Br Med J.* 1999; 518:1280–3.
8. Kopp S, Seestedt-Stanford L, Rohlfing K, et al. Creating adaptive environments. *Planning Higher Ed.* 2004;32:12–23.
9. Barbour A. *Group Methods and Affective Learning.* Report No. CS 509 927. Denver, CO: University of Denver School of Communications; 1998. ERIC Document Reproduction Service No. ED 424 599.
10. Pierce J, Kalkman D. Applying learner-centered principles in teacher education. *Theory Into Prac.* 2003;(42)2:127–32.
11. Zophy, J. On learner-centered teaching. The Scholarly Journal Archive (JSTOR). www.jstor.org.novacat.nova.edu/jstore/gifcvtdir/ap001332/00182745. Accessed June 13, 2004.

People who strive to learn throughout their lifetime have high standards, ambitious goals, and a genuine sense of mission in their lives. Their goals and aspirations spur them on.

John P. Kotter

Developing Lifelong Learning Habits

Fred M. Eckel

Objectives

- Appreciate the need for congruity in words and actions.
- Understand the place of wisdom and expertise in student development.
- Provide tools to develop lifelong learning skills.

Once a student appreciates the obligation of professionals to be competent, you have initiated the first step in the commitment to lifelong learning. Some suggest that professionals serve at the pleasure of society to meet needs society cannot meet for itself. As pharmacists and preceptors, when we interpret our responsibility as an obligation to patients to do what is best for them, we are forced to think about how to maintain professional competence throughout our career. During the experiential training period, when students are more open to learning, the preceptor has the best opportunity to inculcate values that will establish a lifelong commitment to learning, practice growth, and change. Although talking about this obligation to lifelong learning is important, it is more important that the preceptor model the commitment. As preceptors, when our own words and actions are consistent, we have a powerful tool to positively influence our students. Our actions are much more powerful than our words. But when there is congruency between them, the impact may be life changing to students.

As a resident I was fortunate to have a preceptor who modeled consistency between his words and actions. Forty years later I am still reminded of the lessons I learned in my residency. The principles, attitudes, and obligations I was taught are still prominent in my thoughts today. This perspective (principles, attitudes, obligations) is the professional wisdom of what preceptors can convey to students in those teachable moments that occur frequently during an experiential training program. Think of professional wisdom as learning that occurs when knowledge is combined with experience to enable the learner to understand the underlying principle of a particular situation. Wisdom allows us to do the right thing rather than just do things right. The attainment of professional wisdom is what separates the expert from the competent professional. The expert does the right thing while the competent practitioner does things right. The profession of pharmacy needs more experts.

When preceptors instill lifelong learning skills into their students, they begin the process that can lead students toward becoming experts. The trainees must continue learning and reflecting to become experts. As preceptors, we can facilitate the process, perhaps we can even jump-start it as we share our wisdom, but, ultimately, students must make the commitment to lifelong learning if they expect to become experts.

Clifton J. Latiolais, my preceptor, was responsible for starting my career by sharing his wisdom. His contributions to pharmacy are legendary. He served as president of several pharmacy associations, and his practice innovations were duplicated in many settings. His greatest contribution was the practitioners he mentored, who themselves became practice leaders and innovators. He in-

◆ **PRECEPTOR PEARLS**

Some ideas to help facilitate teaching lifelong learning to students:

1. *We reproduce what we are.* People cannot give to others what they themselves do not possess. To teach lifelong learning skills you have to practice lifelong learning. Remember, we teach what we know and we reproduce what we are.
2. *If you want to continue developing as a preceptor, you need to keep learning from others.* You can learn the foundational skills to precept from other pharmacists, but your effectiveness will be increased as you learn precepting skills from preceptors in many professions.

(continued, page 16)

(continued from page 15)

3. *Prepare daily for your next position.* Someone once suggested to me that you should spend a little time each day preparing for your next position.

   I have found this suggestion an important contribution lifelong learning. A caution, however, is that if you spend too much effort on preparing for your next job that you do a poor job in your current position, then you might not have the opportunity to be considered for another position. Becoming involved in a pharmacy organization is one way to develop skills and insights to prepare for your next professional opportunity. Therefore, a preceptor should encourage students to get involved in pharmacy organizations while in school and during their experiential rotations. Making time for that involvement sets an example that will be valuable for a lifetime.

4. *Precept your students throughout their career.* Personal and professional development involve a lifetime of effort.

   A special relationship often develops between a preceptor and students. When the preceptor recognizes this unique opportunity he or she has to influence, he or she will realize the possibility of continuing that influence on their protégés, if the preceptor follows up with the students over time. Ev-

stilled in us a commitment to lifelong learning. Because he was able to multiply the influence of his ideas through the leaders he mentored, he has left a legacy within the profession. More than modeling his personal commitment to lifelong learning, as a preceptor he also instilled this same commitment in his students, which is why he was able to influence and reproduce such a large number of practice leaders. Throughout my career I wanted to live up to the standards my mentor instilled in me. He helped me love change, strive for excellence, and enjoy being a pharmacist. I will always be indebted to him for the role he had in my life. I have strived to give back to others an appreciation for what he did for me personally and professionally.

ery time I interacted professionally with my preceptor long after my training was completed, he taught me something or held me accountable for my professional contributions. He was always my mentor. He did not feel like he graduated from the responsibility, and I continue to benefit from his insights throughout my career. For continuous learning to occur you need to recognize you can learn from everyone, but when your preceptor commits to your continued learning throughout your career, your lifelong learning is enhanced. As a preceptor I hope you do this for your students.

5. *Reflection is an important component of lifelong learning.* Unless we take the time to think about what happened each day we lose the opportunity to really learn from our experiences. Reflection is how we gain wisdom.

   Reflection is not practiced very well in our culture, which values action instead of contemplation. Maintaining a learning diary each day is an effective tool for reflection and teaching. In spare minutes during the day, write down key things you have learned. At the end of the day, add together the three major experiences of the day. From this you can prepare action plans based on what you have learned. As your students collect these insights throughout their experiential rotation, they will have assembled a set of action plans to guide them throughout their career. The habit of reflection will assure that your students will engage in lifelong learning.

What lies behind us and what lies before us are tiny matters compared to what lies within us.

Ralph Waldo Emerson

Developing Workplace Skills

Traci L. Metting

Objectives

- Describe the importance of workplace skills.
- List and give examples of the Four Cs skills.

Workplace skills are essential to any practitioner in his or her career. Developing workplace skills is often like buying a diamond: you look for the characteristic Four Cs—cut, color, clarity, and carat—to determine quality.[1] Students are diamonds in the rough, and the Four Cs of communication, compassion, cooperation, and confidence are critical in the success of these students.[2] Students work to develop these characteristics as they proceed through their education, but the true test comes when these skills have been put to use and didactic knowledge is applied.

Much like diamonds, as students progress through their training, different pressures are applied. If the amount of pressure and the chemistry are right, a mass of carbon atoms will end as a brilliant, multifaceted diamond. The same can be said about pharmacy students. It is under the guidance of the master craftsman (preceptor) that these skills are shaped; the rough edges are shaped into smooth facets, and as the students make the transition to practitioners, a beautiful diamond represents the best of what the master jeweler has created. As the master jeweler, it is the job of the preceptor to work with the students to develop these characteristics.

Communication

Advances in technology have changed the way we communicate. Letter writing has been replaced by short, succinct responses via e-mail. As a result, many organizations have experienced potentially damaging breakdowns in communication. To prevent this, it is imperative that we train our students to be good communicators.

Communication has two main parts: the sender's message, and the interpretation of this message by the receiver. This would appear to be relatively simple, but if you have ever played the childhood game of telephone, you know that many messages end up differently than originally intended. What causes the game of telephone to be exciting is the fact that this message is often clouded by external noise.

External noise can come in many forms, including the choice of words that are used, body language, assumptions, perceptual biases, existing relationships between the communicators, and cultural differences. As the message comes through this noise, it is often distorted, resulting in a message that is miscommunicated. As the decibel level of the environmental noise grows, there is more room for miscommunication.

It is the job of the preceptor to work with the students to facilitate an understanding of good communication. The students should be given ample opportunities to work on building their communication skills through practicing communication in diverse situations. Examples of ways to practice both verbal and written communication skills with students include the following:

- Patient counseling.
- Creating educational presentations for the staff.
- Writing the answers to drug information questions.
- Preparing drug information sheets or patient education handouts.
- Role playing with the students, factoring in environmental noise.
- Experience. There is no better teacher than experience. Allow the students every opportunity to practice communication. If you witness a breakdown in communication, work with the students to address ways in which the communication could have gone differently. If you are involved in a miscommunication that could serve as a learning experience for the students, tell the students about it and let them learn from your experience. Once a basic understanding of effective communication and the barriers to it are obtained, students will begin to master an essential workplace skill.

Compassion

Compassion is an essential skill in health care. Being able to put yourself in the position of the patient requires a skill that some students do not have. Many times, instead of compassion, students display pity or apathy for the patient. This is detrimental to both the students and the patient and keeps them from having a beneficial relationship. Students should be taught that compassion involves understanding the suffering of others and doing something to help decrease or eliminate the patient's suffering.

Preceptors should encourage students to become involved in a patient's care and not limit their interactions to only those things pertaining to the practice of pharmacy. Instead, the students should be involved not only with the patient's health as it relates to medication but also with the patient's spiritual, mental, and social health. By empowering students to become involved with issues that are facing the patient, students will develop a sense of compassion and responsibility for the patient. Both students and their patients will benefit from this interaction.

To help students learn to develop compassion,

- have them take on a challenging patient with complex psychosocial issues.
- identify a special-needs patient (deaf, hard of hearing, mentally challenged, or blind) and have students spend time counseling the patient on his or her medications.
- have students spend a day with case management or social services so they gain a better understanding of the challenges facing patients.
- in areas where there are opportunities to do so (a nursing home or pediatric unit), allow students to interact with the patients on a social level. An example of this is letting the students play bingo with a group of patients in a nursing home.

Taking time to understand more about patients and their needs will help students develop the capacity for compassion. In addition, this interaction will enable students to be accepting and to have compassion for the patients they encounter.

Cooperation

Alexander Graham Bell said, "Great discoveries and improvements invariably involve the cooperation of many minds." Bell's invention of the telephone lends support to this statement by recognizing that we have to have easy communication between parties in order to get a task accomplished. Knowing this, it is easy to see why the ability to cooperate is critical in the workplace. Cooperation involves working together to reach an agreed-on endpoint, which refers back to developing teamwork skills.

It is critical for students to develop teamwork. We learn from an early age to play well with others. However, the real challenges arise when we have to play successfully in a group in which we might not agree with the others.

Teams are made up of many different combinations of people all having different needs, strengths, and ideas. It is important that students learn that in any team there will be natural leaders, followers, entrepreneurs, dissenters, and devil's advocates. All of the members will play an essential role in the productivity of the team, and it is acceptable for the team not to agree 100% of the time. Many times, the compromises a team must make produce the best outcomes.

To help students learn about cooperation and teamwork, they should be given the opportunity to

- work as a member of a particular team.
- lead a team to find a solution to a common problem.
- work with teams that are made up of different types of people (patients, nurses, physicians, or other health care providers).
- work in a small, controlled group and assume different roles in the group (leader, devil's advocate, etc.).

Confidence

Peter T. McIntyre said, "Confidence comes not from always being right but from not fearing to be wrong." Gaining confidence is often the most difficult skill to achieve because it has to be acquired. Confidence is also very hard for a preceptor to teach because many preceptors do not have the confidence they need themselves. As with a practitioner, a student's confidence will increase with each success. How these successes and failures are addressed plays a critical role in shaping the confidence of the students.

The best thing you can do for students is to set them up to succeed. One good way to do this is to have students work on a question that needs to be answered. While the students are working on the answer, ask questions and guide them through any thought processes that might be missing. Next, have students present the original question and their answer to you. After the presentation of the information, ask students what questions they would want answered if they were requesting the information. Then ask the students questions that you have about the information. If the students stumble over the answers, walk them through the thought process involved in answering the question. When the students have a good grasp of the information and potential questions that might be asked, allow them to present the answer to the person who initially requested the information. The preparation will build the students' confidence and a successful presentation will solidify that confidence. After the presentation, the preceptor should debrief the students. Constructive comments should be given regarding what the students could have improved on, and areas of excellence should be highlighted. Always remember that confidence is shaped not only by successes but also by the ways in which failures are handled. Turning bad experiences into learning experiences will help build the students' confidence.

Students come to us as diamonds in the rough. It is the job of the preceptor to be the master craftsman, assuring that the students that are produced are diamonds. By ensuring that the four workplace skills of communication, compassion, cooperation, and confidence are achieved, we are assuring the quality of the students. Every student has the potential to be a diamond through successful acquisition of these skills.

References

1. DeBeers. The 4Cs of measuring quality. Available at: http://www.DeBeers.com. Accessed June 9, 2004.
2. Gates A, Della-Piana C, Bernat A. Affinity groups: a framework for developing workplace skills. Frontiers in Education Clearinghouse. Available at: http://fie.engrng.pitt.edu/fie97/papers/1113.pdf. Accessed June 9, 2004.

In civilized life, law floats in a sea of ethics.

Earl Warren

Chapter 3

Law and Ethics in Experiential Training

Diane B. Ginsburg, Vikki Jill Polk

Chapter Outline

Pharmacy Rules and Regulations: State Board of Pharmacy Requirements for Preceptors

Vikki Jill Polk, Diane B. Ginsburg

Objectives

- Define the term *preceptor* as boards of pharmacy use it.
- Describe the procedures for pharmacists to become preceptors within their respective states.
- Describe the general authority of boards of pharmacy as they relate to experiential training programs.

A preceptor plays a significant role in the training and development of future pharmacist practitioners. The term *preceptor* is defined by most state boards of pharmacy as follows: a pharmacist licensed in the state to practice pharmacy who meets the preceptor requirements specified by rules and who is certified by the board to supervise pharmacist interns. Most states mandate that for pharmacist interns to count hours worked in a pharmacy, they must be under the direct supervision of a pharmacist who is certified as a preceptor. This requirement does not necessarily apply to hours that students must complete to satisfy degree requirements of their respective academic program. It is not uncommon for pharmacist interns to complete a rotation during their experiential program and be supervised by a physician or other health care provider.

For certification as a preceptor, most states require that a pharmacist be licensed and have at least one year of experience in his/her respective practice setting. Some states recognize pharmacy residency program training and allow pharmacy residents to apply for preceptor certification during their residency (e.g., Texas will allow a pharmacist who has been in an American Society of Health-System Pharmacists (ASHP) accredited residency for at least six months to serve as a preceptor if all other requirements are met).

Most states require some form of preceptor education as part of the initial certification process. To maintain preceptor status, preceptors are required to complete additional hours of preceptor-specific education to maintain their certification. In some states, this continuing education is tied to the licensure renewal cycle. Some colleges require that preceptors complete continuing education specific to their program prior to their certification as preceptors. Many colleges and schools offer annual preceptor education conferences as well as partnering with state professional associations to provide preceptor training.

Each state has its own requirements regarding the ratio of preceptors to interns. Most states limit this ratio to one-to-one in direct patient care activities. In some states, colleges of pharmacy may apply for an exemption to this rule to allow for an expansion of the ratio. The ratios do not usually apply to nontraditional practice settings or in situations where the hours completed by an intern are for satisfying degree requirements rather than for licensure.

The supervision and teaching of future practitioners is a large responsibility for preceptors. The purpose of the internship program is for students to learn the proper way to practice pharmacy and abide by all laws and rules that govern pharmacy practice. Licenses must be in good standing in order for pharmacists to supervise pharmacy students. Unfortunately, things can happen in a pharmacy that can result in disciplinary action against the pharmacy and/or pharmacist's license even if they were not directly responsible. Even though there may not have been any malicious intent on the part of the pharmacist preceptor, a pharmacy and pharmacist that are the subject of a board-imposed penalty should not precept students until the disciplinary action has been resolved and the licenses have been returned to good standing. Some states do allow pharmacists to petition the board to have their preceptor certification reinstated at an earlier time. In this case, it is up to the individual board of pharmacy to render this discussion. Pharmacy board requirements for preceptors by state are listed in Table 3.1.

Licensure

Licensure is not a section in Table 3.1 since pharmacists are required to be licensed by the board or regulatory agent of the particular state in which they will be serving as preceptors. Every state listed in Table 3.1 has deemed pharmacists as preceptors because they are licensed pharmacists and have met the other requirements. Most often it is noted that the pharmacist must be in

Table 3.1 • *Board of Pharmacy Requirements for Preceptors*

State	Credentials	Length of Practice	Complete Application	Approval/ Certified	Training Seminar	Legal Standing
Alabama[1]		2 y	Yes	Approval	Yes	
Alaska[2]	Yes					
Arizona*[3]		1 y		Approval		Yes
Arkansas*[4]		>2 y	Yes	Certified		Yes
California[5]						Yes
Colorado*[6]		2 y	Yes	Both		5 y
Connecticut[7]						
Delaware[8]		2 y				
D.C.*[9]						
Florida[10]	Yes	2 y			Yes	Yes
Georgia[11]						
Hawaii[12]						
Idaho[13]	Yes					
Illinois[14]						
Indiana*[15]				Approval		
Iowa[16]						
Kansas[17]		2 y		Approval		
Kentucky*[18]		1 y				
Louisiana[19]	Yes	2 y	Yes	Certified	Yes	Yes
Maine[20]						
Maryland*[21]	Yes			Approval		Yes
Massachusetts[22]		1 y		Approval		
Michigan[23]		1 y	Yes	Approval		5 y
Minnesota[24]		4,000 h	Yes		Yes	
Mississippi[25]						
Missouri[26]						
Montana[27]		2 y	Yes	Approval		3 y
Nebraska[28]						
Nevada[29]						
New Hampshire[30]						
New Jersey[31]		2 y	Yes	Certified		Yes
New Mexico[32]		1 y		Certified		Yes
New York[33]						
North Carolina*[34]						Yes
North Dakota[35]						
Ohio[36]						
Oklahoma*[37]	Yes	1 y	Yes	Certified		Yes
Oregon[38]		1 y	Yes	Approval		
Pennsylvania[39]			Yes			Yes

Table 3.1 • *Board of Pharmacy Requirements for Preceptors (continued)*

State	Credentials	Length of Practice	Complete Application	Approval/ Certified	Training Seminar	Legal Standing
Rhode Island[40]						
South Carolina[41]						
South Dakota[42]			*Yes*			
Tennessee[43]						
Texas[44]		*1 y*	*Yes*	*Both*	*Yes*	*Yes*
Utah[*45]		*2 y*	*Yes*			
Vermont[46]		*1 y*		*Approval*		
Virginia[47]						
Washington[48]	*Yes*	*1 y*		*Certified*	*Yes*	*Yes*
West Virginia[49]	*Yes*					
Wisconsin[50]						
Wyoming[51]		*2 y*	*Yes*	*Both*		

References

1. Alabama: http://www.albop.com/.
2. Alaska: http://www.dced.state.ak.us/occ/pub/PharmacyStatutes.pdf 12ACC 52.220.
3. Arizona: http://www.pharmacy.state.az.us/R301-305.htm.
4. Arkansas: http://www.state.ar.us/asbp/ and http://www.arkansas.gov/asbp/pdf/lawbook03/REGULATION_02_Nov03.pdf 02-01-0005.
5. California: http://www.pharmacy.ca.gov/intern_preceptor_manual.htm#appendix_c California Code of Regulations, Chapter 17, Title 16, Section 1726, http://www.pharmacy.ca.gov/rph_licensee.htm#preceptor.
6. Colorado: http://www.dora.state.co.us/pharmacy/PhaLicRqmts.htm and http://www.dora.state.co.us/pharmacy/Forms/PreceptorAppl.pdf.
7. Connecticut: http://www.ctdrugcontrol.com/druglaws903.htm Sec. 20-576-8.
8. Delaware: http://professionallicensing.state.de.us/boards/pharmacy/documents/PRACTICAL_EXPERIENCE_PROGRAM_FOR_PHARMACY_PRECEPTORS_AND_INTERNS.doc.
9. District of Columbia: http://dchealth.dc.gov/prof_license/services/pdffile/PDF_frameset.asp?strAppId=15&id=pharmacy/MunicipalPharmacistsRegulations.pdf 6511.
10. Florida: Garnet Keller Program Operations Administrator. [e-mail information from Rule 64B16-26.401]. Florida Board of Pharmacy & Nursing Home Administrators; January 21, 2004.
11. Georgia: http://www.sos.state.ga.us/acrobat/examboards/pharmacy/intern_2002.pdf. and Thompson R. [e-mail]. I&R Specialists; January 20, 2004.
12. Hawaii: http://www.hawaii.gov/dcca/pdf/pvl_pharmacist_exam.pdf.
13. Idaho: http://www3.state.id.us/cgi-bin/newidst?sctid=540170005.K and http://www3.state.id.us/cgi-bin/newidst?sctid=540170022.K.
14. Illinois: Administrative Rules, Section 1330.20 (a-f): http://www.legis.state.il.us/commission/jcar/admincode/068/068013300000200R.html.
15. Indiana: http://www.ai.org/hpb/boards/isbp/2003_lawbook_complete.doc.
16. Iowa: http://www.state.ia.us/ibpe/pharmacists/preceptor.html.
17. Kansas: http://www.accesskansas.org/pharmacy/ce.html.

Table 3.1 • *Board of Pharmacy Requirements for Preceptors (continued)*

18. Kentucky: http://www.state.ky.us/boards/pharmacy/license_renewal.htm.
19. Louisiana: http://www.labp.com/, § 513.
20. Maine: ftp://ftp.state.me.us/pub/sos/cec/rcn/apa/02/392/392c010.doc. Chapter 10, Sec. 6.
21. Maryland: MacCubbin, D. [e-mail]. College Park, MD: University of Maryland School of Pharmacy; January 22, 2004.
22. Massachusetts: http://www.state.ma.us/reg/boards/ph/cmr/24702.htm.
23. Michigan: http://www.state.mi.us/orr/emi/admincode.asp?AdminCode=Single&Admin_Num=33800471&Dpt=CI&RngHigh=, R 338.473c.
24. Minnesota: http://www.phcybrd.state.mn.us/forms/preceptorapp.pdf.
25. Mississippi: http://www.mbp.state.ms.us/.
26. Missouri: http://www.moga.state.mo.us/statutes/C300-399/3380000035.HTM.
27. Montana: http://www.discoveringmontana.com/dli/bsd/license/bsd_boards/pha_board/rules.asp#6.
28. Nebraska: Curtis-Beard, C. [e-mail]. January 27, 2004.
29. Nevada: http://www.leg.state.nv.us/NRS/NRS-639.html.
30. New Hampshire: http://www.gencourt.state.nh.us/rsa/html/XXX/318/318-18.htm.
31. New Jersey: http://www.state.nj.us/lps/ca/pharm/pharmacy.pdf.
32. New Mexico: http://www.state.nm.us/pharmacy/part5.html.
33. New York: http://assembly.state.ny.us/leg/?cl=30&a=132.
34. North Carolina: http://www.ncbop.org/SummaryOfStandards.htm and Stump, D. [phone conversation]. February 2, 2004.
35. North Dakota: http://www.nodakpharmacy.com/NDBP/law/lawbook_Dec2003.pdf.
36. Ohio: http://pharmacy.ohio.gov/intrnshp-030201.htm.
37. Oklahoma: http://www.state.ok.us/~pharmacy/lawbook.pdf.
38. Oregon: http://www.pharmacy.state.or.us/rules/div031.pdf.
39. Pennsylvania: http://www.pacode.com/secure/data/049/chapter27/chap27toc.html.
40. Rhode Island: http://www.health.ri.gov/hsr/professions/Intern_LimitedLicense.pdf.
41. South Carolina: http://www.scstatehouse.net/code/t40c043.htm.
42. South Dakota: http://legis.state.sd.us/rules/rules/2051.htm#20:51:02:11.
43. Tennessee: http://www.state.tn.us/sos/rules/1140/1140-02.pdf.
44. Texas: http://www.tsbp.state.tx.us/files_Word/CERT-PRECEPTOR.doc.
45. Utah: http://www.dopl.utah.gov/licensing/forms/011.doc.
46. Vermont: http://vtprofessionals.org/opr1/pharmacists/forms/rxrules.pdf.
47. Virginia: http://www.dhp.state.va.us/pharmacy/leg/Pharmacy%20Law%202003.doc.
48. Washington State: http://www.leg.wa.gov/wac/index.cfm?fuseaction=Section&Section=246-858-060.
49. West Virginia: http://www.wvbop.com/law1.htm.
50. Wisconsin: http://www.drl.state.wi.us/Regulation/applicant_information/PharmacyPDFs/FAQsPharmacyInternship.pdf.
51. Wyoming: http://soswy.state.wy.us/RULES/4954.pdf.

good standing. Colorado and several other states do not require preceptors in the areas of drug research within a pharmacy school or industry to be licensed pharmacists. Preceptors must be licensed in the state in which they are practicing according to the State Board of Pharmacy in Iowa. An exception to this would be pharmacists practicing in federal facilities who are only required to have a current license in at least one state. Pharmacists practicing in any of the military branches, the Veteran's Administration, or the Bureau of Prisons are only required to be licensed in one state and may practice pharmacy in any facility regardless of location. Federal laws, not individual state laws, have jurisdiction in these facilities.

Credentials

Some states have qualifications or credentials that pharmacists must meet in order to become preceptors. Oklahoma has requirements and qualifications listed under section 535:25-3 of the state pharmacy law book that are used at a minimum to help determine if pharmacists can be preceptors.

Length of Practice

Most states require a specific length of pharmacy practice before pharmacists can precept students. This length of experience is typically the year(s) immediately before becoming a preceptor. Arkansas requires the length of practice to be the two years immediately prior to applying, and the Louisiana State Board of Pharmacy requires that the two years of practice be consecutive years. Minnesota requires that pharmacists practice 4,000 hours before becoming a preceptor, and 2,000 of the 4,000 hours must be in the state of Minnesota.

Complete Application

A state will require pharmacists to complete an application before they can be considered preceptors. These forms are typically located on the website of the board or regulatory agent. This application usually registers pharmacists as preceptors for the particular state in which they are applying.

Approval/Certified

The board of pharmacy or regulatory agent of a state will grant preceptor approval to pharmacists who meet the requirements needed to precept students. Some states require certification to become preceptors, and some states require pharmacists to be both approved and certified. Indiana can approve practical experience supervisors for students, or pharmacists must supervise students. In Louisiana, the certification expires five years after the date of issue, but it can be renewed at the time of application. Louisiana preceptors must "conspicuously display the certification at the primary preceptor pharmacy location." This is common in several states. New Mexico pharmacy preceptors who will be supervising students in another state must be approved from the students' state board of pharmacy to be preceptors. Oklahoma's certification is valid for three years, after which pharmacists must take an exam and pay a fee set by the board. This fee is less than the fee that is required for initial certification. Oklahoma requires that the preceptor certificates be "conspicuously posted in the training area where they practice." Texas also requires certificates to be publicly displayed.

Training Seminar

Some states will have a required board-approved preceptor-training seminar for applicants. These seminars are required for initial approval and then as often as the state deems it necessary to meet requirements. Alabama requires seminar attendance once every three years. Texas requires attendance of a three-hour training program "developed by a Texas college of pharmacy and provided by an ACPE approved provider within the previous two years." Attendance of this training program must be completed again when pharmacists' current licenses are to be renewed. Washington pharmacists must complete their training program within the last five years before applying to become preceptors.

Legal Standing

Legal standing refers to either the specific time period of law observance or if law observance was noted for a particular state. Pharmacist must be in compliance with the law and must not have violated any laws or statutes related to the practice of pharmacy. The Arizona State Board of Pharmacy requires that a pharmacist must have an unrestricted pharmacist's license and must "enter into an agreement satisfactory to the Board that places restrictions on the pharmacist's license if the pharmacist has been found guilty of violating any federal or state law relating to the practice of pharmacy, drug or device distribution or record keeping, or unprofessional conduct." Colorado's State Board of Pharmacy allows an exception if there is a "Letter of Admonition." In Colorado, if a pharmacist has been licensed for less than five years, then the length of law observance must be the length of the pharmacist's license.

Unique Requirements

The Arizona State Board of Pharmacy requires that a pharmacist either be approved by the board or hold a faculty position that is part of the experiential training program of an approved college or school of pharmacy. The Arkansas State Board of Pharmacy requires a pharmacist to "be a full-time pharmacist in a pharmacy which currently holds a Class A rating indicated by the 'Inspection Sheet' for pharmacists outlined by the State Board of Pharmacy." The applicant must also complete a preceptor requirements and responsibilities test that was developed and administered by the board or board representatives. It is required that one preceptor from an intern site be a member of an "appropriate" national pharmaceutical organization. Each Arkansas individual preceptor is required to be a member of a professional state organization and attend one professional meeting during the previous calendar year. Regulation 01-00-0007 specifies fees that are required during the renewal process that takes place every two years and requires a new application.

In the District of Columbia, pharmacists wanting to be preceptors must take the "Oath of Preceptor," which is as follows:

> *I submit that I shall answer all questions concerning the training of a pharmacy intern under my supervision truthfully to the best of my knowledge and belief and that the training I provide will be predominately related to the practice of pharmacy as required by law.*

Pharmacists wanting to be board-approved preceptors in Indiana must include "a detailed description of the proposed practical experience program with respect to time, place, duties, responsibilities, and supervision; and the name of the person responsible for supervising the experience." To be preceptors in Kentucky, pharmacists must submit a written request as well as pay a fee. In Maryland, there is currently one pharmacy school, and the board of pharmacy will periodically review preceptors and assure that the pharmacists are in good moral standing.[1] In North Carolina, if preceptors supervise at least 400 hours of intern experience, the board will grant them five hours of continuing education credits.

Oklahoma requires pharmacists to take a preceptor exam that is prepared by the board relating to subchapter 535:10-5-8 "Preceptor Requirements" as well as pharmacy laws and rules. Verbal examination is also part of the application process to be certified preceptors in Oklahoma. Utah applicants must provide proof of meeting the requirements for continuing education for the two years prior to license renewal. "Applicants must also subscribe to and abide by the Code of Ethics of the American Pharmaceutical Association."*

Summary

The requirements for pharmacists to become preceptors vary from state to state. Being a licensed pharmacist is the only criterion that each state has in common. Table 3.1 makes it apparent that some states have highly structured procedures that are expected of pharmacists wanting to become preceptors. Fourteen percent of the states have specific credentials set in place that are expected of pharmacists before they become preceptors. Only 43% have length of practice experience predetermined for pharmacists, and the length of practice is typically between one to two years. Twenty-nine percent of the states have an actual application form and process established for preceptor applicants, and 35% will approve and/or certify preceptors for the experiential training of interns. Training seminars seem to be the minority approach for state requirements for preceptors. Training seminars are currently being utilized by close to 10% of the states listed. Finally, most state boards of pharmacy and regulatory agents are not citing adherence to legal responsibilities as a requirement for preceptor applicants. This is an area that only about 27% of the states actually listed document observation of law observance in their require-

---

*This application was revised on June 11,2001 and does not reflect the 2003 name change of the American Pharmaceutical Association to the American Pharmacists Association.

ments. Most states will list "good standing with the Board" after licensure requirements, and this can often be interpreted as good legal compliance with the rules and regulations of the state's pharmacy law. However, it is best to give an exact legal compliance time frame, so that expectations are clearly projected.

Reference

1. Good moral character – "A pattern of behavior conforming to a profession's ethical standards and showing an absence of moral turpitude. Good moral character is usually a requirement of persons applying to practice a profession such as law or medicine." Garner, BA. *Black's Law Dictionary.* Abridged 7th ed. St. Paul, MN: West Group; 2000:556.

Liability Issues for Preceptors

Diane B. Ginsburg

Objective

- Discuss liability issues for preceptors.

The training of future pharmacists is a rewarding experience for most preceptors. Students are eager after many years of training to function as licensed practitioners and provide direct patient care. Many students, when they enter the final year of their program, are very mature and appear ready to undertake the responsibilities of licensed pharmacists. The important thing to remember is that although they may seem ready to function as licensed practitioners, they are not licensed. The responsibility of all student actions rests with the preceptor's license.

Most colleges of pharmacy understand the huge responsibility that preceptors have when they are supervising students. Preceptors not only have to worry about their actions (and in some cases, the actions of their staff if they are the pharmacist-in-charge or in a supervisory role), but they also have to worry about the actions of their students.

> **◆ PRECEPTOR PEARLS**
>
> During orientation at the beginning of the rotation, preceptors should
> - ask to see students' proof of liability insurance.
> - discuss the differences between "pharmacist duties" and "intern duties."
> - review procedures for checking students' work.
> - acknowledge students' desire to be of assistance and not a hindrance to providing direct patient care.
> - remind students that you (as their preceptor) are *ultimately responsible* for everything they do and that your license could be disciplined for failure to be in compliance with appropriate laws and rules.

Most students do not intentionally try to make an error; however, the nature of their learning process lends itself to the fact that students are going to make mistakes. Preceptors are ultimately responsible for any errors made by students. This reinforces the importance of checking all work completed by students.

Most programs require that students purchase liability insurance prior to starting their rotations. These policies, which range between $10–$20, only cover activities that the students perform. These policies are not the same as the malpractice insurance that most licensed pharmacists carry.

Ethical Aspects of Precepting Students

Diane B. Ginsburg

Objective

- Review the Code of Ethics for Pharmacists and how it applies to experiential training.

The practice of pharmacy is governed by a strict Code of Ethics. This Code that has been endorsed by virtually all facets of pharmacy, reflects the nature of practice today, a cooperative relationship between pharmacists, other health care providers, and patients. As pharmacists, we think of ethics and this Code as the way pharmacy should be practiced and for most of us, this is the way we practice. It is shocking to think that there are practitioners out there who are both unethical and immoral. The preceptor role is multifold. Preceptors are teachers, mentors, coaches, references, and role models. The future of the profession, our students, looks up to us for guidance, information, and to mirror our actions. These reasons reinforce the importance of ethical behavior and a review of the Code that governs our practice.

Many students remember reciting the Code of Ethics during the white coat ceremony that is usually held during new student orientation. As novices they blindly recite the words, not truly understanding the significance behind them. Many will not think to pull out this document until something happens and they are reminded of this Code. As preceptors, it is essential that students see you "walk your talk" and uphold and abide by this Code. An excellent discussion to have with your students is to review and discuss what the Code of Ethics means to you as a pharmacist and how you demonstrate this in your practice.

Code of Ethics for Pharmacists[1]

"PREAMBLE

Pharmacists are health professionals who assist individuals in making the best use of medications. This Code, prepared and supported by pharmacists, is intended to state publicly the principles that form the fundamental basis of the roles and responsibilities of pharmacists. These principles, based on moral obligations and virtues, are established to guide pharmacists in relationships with patients, health professionals, and society.

I. A pharmacist respects the covenantal relationship between the patient and pharmacist.

Considering the patient-pharmacist relationship as a covenant means that a pharmacist has moral obligations in response to the gift of trust received from society. In return for this gift, a pharmacist promises to help individuals achieve optimum benefit from their medications, to be committed to their welfare, and to maintain their trust.

II. A pharmacist promotes the good of every patient in a caring, compassionate, and confidential manner.

A pharmacist places concern for the well being of the patient at the center of professional practice. In doing so, a pharmacist considers needs stated by the patient as well as those defined by health science. A pharmacist is dedicated to protecting the dignity of the patient. With a caring attitude and a compassionate spirit, a pharmacist focuses on serving the patient in a private and confidential manner.

III. A pharmacist respects the autonomy and dignity of each patient.

A pharmacist promotes the right of self-determination and recognizes individual self-worth by encouraging patients to participate in decisions about their health. A pharmacist communicates with patients in terms that are understandable. In all cases, a pharmacist respects personal and cultural differences among patients.

IV. A pharmacist acts with honesty and integrity in professional relationships.

A pharmacist has a duty to tell the truth and to act with conviction of conscience. A pharmacist avoids discriminatory practices, behavior or work conditions that impair professional judgment, and actions that compromise dedication to the best interests of patients.

V. A pharmacist maintains professional competence.

A pharmacist has a duty to maintain knowledge and abilities as new medications, devices, and technologies become available and as health information advances.

◆ **Preceptor Pearls**

- Review the Code of Ethics with your students at the beginning of the rotation. Discuss what it means to you in practice.
- Ask your students, What does the Code mean to them? How will they implement this Code throughout the remainder of their experiential training and in practice?
- "Walk your talk." Let students see that you practice pharmacy in the most ethical manner possible.
- Remember that students represent many differences including cultural, generational, gender, and work ethic.

VI. A pharmacist respects the values and abilities of colleagues and other health professionals.

When appropriate, a pharmacist asks for the consultation of colleagues or other health professionals or refers the patient. A pharmacist acknowledges that colleagues and other health professionals may differ in the beliefs and values they apply to the care of the patient.

VII. A pharmacist serves individual, community, and societal needs.

The primary obligation of a pharmacist is to individual patients. However, the obligations of a pharmacist may at times extend beyond the individual to the community and society. In these situations, the pharmacist recognizes the responsibilities that accompany these obligations and acts accordingly.

VIII. A pharmacist seeks justice in the distribution of health resources.

When health resources are allocated, a pharmacist is fair and equitable, balancing the needs of patients and society."

*Adopted by the membership of the American Pharmacists Association, October 27, 1994.

As important as this Code is to practice, it is equally important that preceptors and their staff treat students with respect and dignity. Many issues come into play when precepting students: demands of the work place, staff needs, knowledge base of the students, and generational differences. Today's students can use automated databases and computers more comfortably than a hard copy textbook. They have been taught drug information in an integrated fashion versus by discipline (e.g., chemistry, pharmacology, clinical application). For some tenured practitioners, this presents both an opportunity and a challenge. The opportunity is one where students can teach preceptors and expose them to the benefits of their education. The challenge for some preceptors is resistance to a new model for pharmacy practice and the way students are being taught.

Reference

1. American Pharmacists Association. *Code of Ethics for Pharmacists.* Washington, DC: American Pharmacists Association; 1997.

Patient Confidentiality and HIPAA

Diane B. Ginsburg

Objective

- Define HIPAA and how it applies to experiential training programs

The issue of patient confidentiality was heightened in lieu of new privacy laws enacted by the federal government. The Health Insurance Portability and Accountability Act (HIPAA) increased the level of due diligence that health care providers are required to exercise to ensure confidentiality of patient protected health information (PHI). Many pharmacies have implemented safeguards and protective measures including training of staff.

> ◆ **Preceptor Pearls**
> - Incorporate HIPAA training as part of your orientation program.
> - Verify your practice site requirements for HIPAA training for students (nonemployees).
> - Verify what type of HIPAA training is conducted at the school and college of pharmacy where you have an affiliation.
> - Incorporate HIPAA and privacy requirements into affiliation agreements with academic institutions.

Most colleges and schools of pharmacy have incorporated HIPAA information in pharmacy jurisprudence courses as part of their discussion of federal law. In addition, HIPAA and privacy issues are discussed prior to the beginning of experiential training for most programs and included in course syllabi for the internship. This does not preclude the HIPAA training requirements of the individual practice site. Students may be expected to complete HIPAA training for each rotation if they are completed at different institutions. A review of HIPAA and privacy rules should be included as part of the orientation to the practice site and conducted during the beginning of the rotation experience.

values, the preceptor must hold each of these values as personally important.

The progression of students from the classroom setting to experiential sites and, ultimately, to professional practice requires personal growth of the students. Students learn to be professionals not from textbooks but rather from observing professionals in the experiential practice setting and functioning as health care providers. The most important person to instill this professionalism in students is the preceptor. To do so, the preceptor must exhibit professional behavior and discuss professional issues with students. The preceptor should also discuss professional organizations with students and encourage students to become active members in professional organizations. Preceptors must be willing to serve as mentors to their students, guiding them along their path from students to pharmacists and helping them move from an educational model of student/teacher to mentor/mentee. (See more on professionalism in chapter 11.) This transition will prepare students for the lifetime learning model that all pharmacists need.

The majority of experiential rotations are supervised by pharmacists who are precepting students while performing their normal duties. Teaching while maintaining a full work schedule requires preceptors to have a true desire to teach and commit the time necessary to teach. These obligations often require preceptors to work overtime. Without the true desire to educate students and the willingness to devote the necessary time, preceptors will not be able to maximize the students' learning experience.

The student population today is more diverse than it was even 10 years ago. This diversity includes ethnic and gender diversity, along with cultural and generational diversity. Many students today are entering pharmacy school after having worked for several years in another profession, and many students today already possess advanced degrees in other fields. While these factors will help strengthen the pharmacy profession in the future, preceptors must recognize and respect these differences. The degree of diversity that exists today also requires preceptors to adapt teaching techniques for maximizing students' learning experiences. When precepting multiple students on the same rotation, diversity factors can present unique and challenging situations.

Technical Skills and Abilities

To be effective, preceptors must be skilled in the work area, have good time management skills, be organized, possess good written and oral communication skills, and understand resource utilization requirements. While strengths in these areas will vary from preceptor to preceptor, preceptors must have some ability in each of these areas.

Precepting students on experiential rotations requires preceptors to have excellent skills in the area that is being taught. If a preceptor is not knowledgeable about a particular area, students will not gain the necessary oversight and guidance to meet their learning objectives. A rotation with an unprepared or inexperienced preceptor can adversely affect the students' view of the profession. Preceptors should never be forced to take students on a rotation if they are not competent in that area. Sometimes—in an effort to schedule an experiential rotation for students—the site will try to accommodate both the students' and college's needs. When this occurs, the site and preceptor almost always fall short, and the result is a derogatory experience for all involved.

As stated above, precepting is an additional duty that a pharmacist takes on because of the desire to be involved in the educational process of our profession. To be effective at balancing the requirements of the job with time spent teaching, preceptors must have good organizational and time management skills. Knowledge of resource utilization requirements of the site is also helpful in achieving this balance, potentially allowing preceptors to work within these resource requirements to involve others in the process.

The purpose of life, after all, is to live it, to task experience to the utmost, to reach out eagerly and without fear for newer and richer experiences.

Eleanor Roosevelt

Necessary Skills to Be an Effective Preceptor

Diane B. Ginsburg, Lee C. Vermeulen

Objectives

- Define the elements of the communication process, and identify the preceptor's role in this process.
- Review the elements of nonverbal communication.
- Describe different questioning and listening techniques to enhance effective interactions between preceptors and students.
- Discuss techniques to teach effective written communication and improve student writing.

Communication Skills

The single most important ability for preceptors is the ability to communicate effectively with students. Students often hear what students want or expect to hear. Effective preceptors will communicate in such a way to ensure that students understand the information that is being presented.

Miscommunication is not limited to the interaction between preceptors and students. Miscommunication happens in all facets of life; however, this can be magnified when trying to teach students. It is easy for preceptors and students to become frustrated many times during experiential training when the objectives and outcomes for a rotation are not clearly stated. When this occurs, the expectations of the preceptors and students are not met, and what should be a positive learning experience quickly disintegrates into a negative experience.

Communication Model

It is important for preceptors to understand how personal communication can

Figure 4-1 • The Interpersonal Communication Model[2]

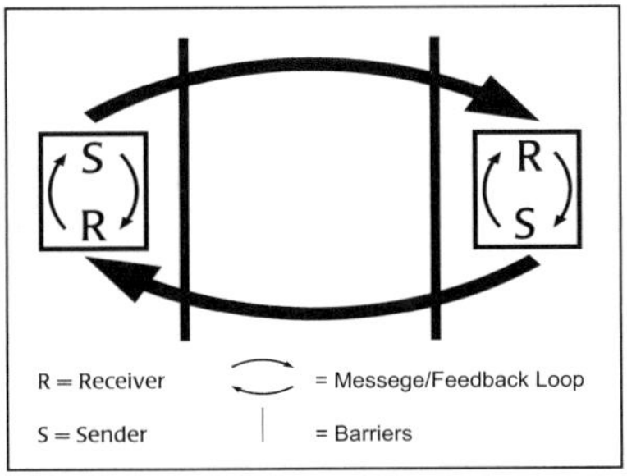

affect their relationship with their students.[1] To be an effective communicator (and hopefully an equally effective preceptor), an understanding of the basic communication model is important. The interpersonal communication model is applicable to all situations, not just to pharmacy practice.

This basic model consists of five main components (Figure 4-1):

- Sender
- Message
- Receiver
- Feedback
- Barriers

Sender

The sender is the one that initiates the communication. This can be done in any setting, face-to-face, over the phone, and via e-mail. In a typical preceptor-student interaction, asking questions of a student would be an example of the preceptor acting as the sender. An example is as follows:

Preceptor: Do you know how frequently patients have hypersensitivity reactions to penicillin antibiotics?
Student: Yes.
***Preceptor* (seeming a little put off by the student's response):** Well, what are they?

In this example it is probably very easy to see why the preceptor was a little irritated with the student's response. The preceptor wanted more than a yes/no response from the student; however, the student answered the exact question asked by the preceptor (did he/she know how frequently reactions occur). The preceptor committed a very common communication sin—asking a closed-ended question and wanting an open-ended question response. When senders ask closed-ended questions, they are limiting the responses of those that receive the information to a one-word answer, usually "yes" or "no." By merely changing the beginning of the question, the preceptor can get the desired response:

Preceptor: How frequently do patients have hypersensitivity reactions to penicillin antibiotics?
Student: Approximately 5–10% of the time.

In the above example, the preceptor changed the question from closed-ended to open-ended by placing *How* at the beginning. An open-ended question is easily accomplished by using one of the five *W* questions or the *H* question: who, what, where, when, why, and how.

We do not realize how common this communication error is and how much miscommunication is caused by asking closed-ended questions and expecting an open-ended response. Preceptors must be conscious of their communication style and manner in which they ask questions. Students coming out of pharmacy programs today are receiving more training in communication skills than was part of the training for many preceptors. Questioning and listening skills are two areas that are covered in didactic and laboratory experiences. Role-playing and feedback from colleagues are two ways in which your questioning style can be evaluated.

Message

The message is the most common place for miscommunication to occur. This is the element that is actually transmitted from one individual to another through various means. In both examples listed above, part of the message was the actual dialog between the preceptor and the student. The question itself was the message the preceptor was trying to send. The manner in which the message is sent can change how it is interpreted or decoded by others.

As with all aspects of the communication process, it is not only what you say but how you say it that can cause a breakdown in communication. As important as the actual words you select, your body language, facial expressions, tone of voice, and inflection are all nonverbal aspects of communication that can cause miscommunication. In most situations, the sender formulates the question before it is transmitted. How it is conveyed and/or expressed is usually where the miscommunication occurs. Examples of nonverbal communications are as follows:

- Facial expressions
- Gestures
- Body language
- Posture
- Eye contact
- Tone of voice and inflection

Characteristics of one's voice are also a nonverbal aspect of communication. The tone of voice one uses can dramatically change the meaning of a message. For example, the following sentence would have two different meanings depending on the tone of voice used:

Pleasant tone: "You did a great job!"
Sarcastic tone: "You did a great job!"

Same wording—two completely different meanings. If a preceptor (sender) used this phrase and changed the tone in which it was delivered when giving feedback on an assignment, it would be easy to see how the student (receiver) could get two different messages. It is very important that you are conscious of the nonverbal elements of the voice in two-way communications.

Receiver

The receiver is the one that receives the message and tries to decode it to determine what is being asked or requested. When communication goes well, this is easy, but when the sender transmits a message saying one thing verbally and another nonverbally, the receiver is at a loss as to what it is the sender wants. This is the proverbial "What did they mean by that?" scenario that is common in communication where the verbal message indicates one thing; however, the nonverbal message indicates something completely different. The following is an example of a two-sided message:

> The student sits down with the preceptor for a mid-rotation evaluation. The conversation goes as follows:
>
> ***Preceptor:*** I have seen significant improvement in your drug information consults since the beginning of the rotation.
> ***Student:*** I am glad to hear that as I have really worked hard on these.
> ***Preceptor (looking somewhat stern):*** You still have some work to do in this area before the end of the rotation.
>
> The student meets with some classmates later that day and tells them that based on what the preceptor said, failing the rotation is inevitable.

What happened in this scenario? The student received feedback from the preceptor regarding performance on a specific task. The preceptor initially indicated that the student had improved; however, the student still had some deficiencies that needed to be worked on prior to the end of the rotation. The student decoded the message to mean that he/she was going to fail the rotation. Although this may seem like an overreaction on the part of the student, this is a common occurrence. The student expected his/her level of improvement to be enough; however, there were still things that needed to be done relating to this activity, and the preceptor was trying to get the point across that there had been improvement. In the preceptor's attempt to indicate that the student still needed to improve, the preceptor came across in a stern manner that the student misunderstood to have another meaning (i.e., that he/she was going to fail the rotation).

This is a classic example of where the message was delivered and decoded differently by the receiver than what the sender intended. In a situation like the one described above, the potential exists for the student to be apprehensive to ask the preceptor for any feedback. The expression "reading into what someone just said" is a common facet of miscommunication. This occurs when there is not congruence between the verbal and nonverbal aspects of the message.

Feedback

Feedback is where the receiver and sender change roles in the communication process. This is the element of the communication model that makes communication a two-way process. The receiver, in response to the message that is transmitted by the sender, communicates back to the sender. This may be an answer to a question or an inquiry in response to a facial expression by the sender. In the communication model, senders and receivers are constantly moving back and forth between the roles of sender and receiver. Feedback is a critical part of the communication process because when used effectively, this is the place where miscommunication can be corrected. Feedback can be both verbal and nonverbal. Sometimes a mere nodding of one's head can indicate to the sender that the receiver understands. In situations where something complex is being discussed, feedback can be used to determine the level of understanding of the receiver. Let's look at the previous scenario with feedback being used by both the preceptor and the student:

Preceptor: I have seen significant improvement in your drug information consults since the beginning of the rotation.

Student: I am glad to hear that as I have really worked hard on these.

Preceptor (looking somewhat stern): You still have some work to do in this area before the end of the rotation.

Student (looking scared): Do you mean that I have not done enough to pass the rotation?

Preceptor: No, that is not what I meant. You have improved quite a bit since the beginning of the rotation; however, there are still some things you need to include in your consults. I am sure as you do a few more throughout the remainder of the rotation that this will improve. I know this is the first rotation where you have had to do this type of writing and you haven't had much experience in this area. Let's sit down the next time you write your next consult so we can go over these things.

Student (looking somewhat relieved): Thank you for the feedback. I appreciate all of your assistance with this.

In the scenario above, feedback cleared up a misconception that the student had regarding the outcome of the rotation. Certainly, the preceptor did not mean to scare the student; however, it is easy to see why the student felt he/she may fail the rotation. It is essential that the verbal and nonverbal messages (whether it is the initial sending of the message or through the feedback loop) are parallel so miscommunication/misinterpretation does not occur.

Barriers

Barriers are anything that prevents effective communication and transmission of the message. Barriers can be physical, such as counters, glass partitions, talking on the phone, e-mail, and other forms of electronic communication, which prevent the receiver and sender to read and decode nonverbal communication. Removal of these physical barriers facilitates feedback and prevents miscommunication.

With electronic communication, such as e-mail messages, this is sometimes difficult as the message is seen as one-dimensional. Selection and use of words can indicate a tone that the sender of the message did not intend. Sending "flaming" messages (e.g., using all capitols, no punctuation, etc.) can give the message a completely different meaning then the sender intended. Without a web cam (which is only minimally effective to facilitate reading nonverbal communications), the only things the receiver can decode are the words and phrasing of the message. To compound this, when the sender does not respond immediately to the receiver's response, the receiver can further read something negative in the message.

Questioning and Listening Skills

Questioning and listening skills go hand-in-hand in effective communication. As discussed previously, the manner in which a question is asked can dictate the type of response (e.g., closed-ended question, one word response). All types of questions need to be incorporated in effective communication including closed-ended, open-ended, leading, and probing questions. Examples of these types of questions are shown in Table 4.1.

The key to getting the desired response is directly related to the type of

Table 4.1 • *Types of Questions*

Closed-ended	*Have you ever prepared a TPN solution?*
Open-ended	*What are your goals for this rotation?*
Leading	*How would you counsel the patient?*
Probing	*What else could be done to minimize the side effect profile of the current regimen?*

question asked. This is important for preceptors and students as miscommunication can and will occur when the wrong type of question is asked. This is a great learning exercise for both parties involved when feedback is incorporated. When feedback is used effectively, either party—sender or receiver—can indicate a level of understanding and use additional questions to elicit the desired information. Good questioning skills take practice and the willingness and awareness of others to provide input.

Listening skills are equally as important as the manner in which a question is asked. Being a good listener is not as easy it seems. Active listening takes focus and desire on the part of the listener. It is easy to be distracted from listening to what others have to say, especially students. Phones, interruptions, and stress are all examples of why even the most conscientious listener stops listening. Frequently we fall into the habit of "selective listening" where we appear to be listening by nodding our heads and mumbling "uh huh," "hmm," and "okay." What happens in the preceptor-student relationship is that the student will cease to ask questions and talk to the preceptor because he/she feels that the preceptor is not listening and is disinterested.

It is very gratifying to be a good listener. Everyone can probably remember a patient that they helped because they took the time to listen. This is a very important skill to demonstrate to students. As mentioned in previous sections, students will mirror the behaviors of their preceptors. This is one skill that all health care providers must learn. When selective listening is incorporated, it is easy to miss crucial information when talking to patients. It is important to remember to listen more than to talk. The following quotation is an excellent reminder of this:

The reason we have two ears and only one mouth, is
that we may hear more and speak less.
Zeno (335 BC–264 BC)

Communication must be clear, concise, and fair. Feedback must be provided to students throughout the rotation experience rather than waiting for the formal evaluation period. Feedback must be provided in such a way that students understand the expectations of the preceptor. Effective feedback provides students the knowledge of what needs to be done, challenging students to improve without destroying the students' sense of accomplishment.

Written Communication Skills

As knowledge-based professionals, pharmacists are dependent on their ability to transfer information to care appropriately for patients. While that transfer of knowledge most often takes place verbally, written communication skills are essential. As noted in recent surveys, written skills are not only needed by pharmacy administrators and educators but, increasingly, are also needed as a prerequisite for successful pharmacy practice in all settings.[3,4] Preceptors must be prepared to provide students with training on effective and efficient writing.

The first step in becoming better at teaching writing skills as a preceptor is recognizing that students seldom appreciate the importance of being good writers! For most students, writing is at best an onerous and distasteful task. Preceptors must emphasize the fact that nothing demonstrates professionalism and competence more quickly than clear, concise, and informative writing. Correspondingly, lack of clarity and expression will quickly compromise a pharmacist's credibility in the eyes of patients and other professionals.

You (and your students!) must also accept the fact that being a good writer is not an attribute that anyone is born with. It is a skill, like any other, that must be taught, practiced, and improved. As a preceptor, you will transfer writing skills passively to your students as they read your written work and recognize the quality of your writing. You must also respond to your students' written documents. Your willingness and ability to provide constructive criticism, by editing rather than simply critiquing their work, will determine the impact you will have on their writing skills. In other words, the most effective means of teaching students to be better writers are writing well and editing their work in a constructive manner.

Pharmacists are expected to write in a wide variety of formats, and preceptors should provide students with exposure to each of the various types of documents common in their practice area. It is useful to contrast differences in style, tone, cadence, and even grammatical form required of various written documents. For example, a particular form of writing is used for written progress notes in patients' medical records that may not necessarily emphasize precise grammar, sentence structure, or even punctuation. In contrast, higher expectations are normally set for new drug monographs written for presentation to Pharmacy and Therapeutics Committees. However, accuracy of information, appropriate use of medical terminology, avoidance of dangerous abbreviations, and correct spelling are important issues regardless of what is being written.

> ◆ **PRECEPTOR PEARLS**
> - Set time aside at the beginning of the rotation to review objectives and expectations of the students.
> - Clarify any questions and/or misconceptions students may have at the beginning of the rotation.
> - Schedule time free of interruptions to meet with your students. This will help facilitate open communication throughout the rotation.
> - Listen, listen, listen!
> - Remember that students are vulnerable and sometimes are hesitant to ask questions. Encourage open dialog so that both preceptor and students can get the most out of the rotation.

Institution-specific style manuals should be developed and provided to students to assist in identifying important writing conventions relevant to particular types of written documents. In the absence of a particular desired format, the *American Medical Association Manual of Style*[5] can serve as a guide for appropriate format, style, tone, and cadence of most technical biomedical writing (including issues such as appropriate citation format, technical terminology, and abbreviation standards). Simply requiring students to read several examples of particular document types will assist them in adopting the appropriate tone and format. One of the most valuable tools for honing writing skills is Strunk and White's *The Elements of Style,*[6] which can be found in print for under $10.00. Originally published in 1918 by William Strunk Jr. at Cornell University, the book has undergone several revisions over the years. The full text of the most recent edition (published in 2000) can also be accessed free-of-charge on the World Wide Web. It is an in indispensable guide to good writing that should be read and reread before any substantial writing is undertaken. A variety of other web-based writing resources can be found as well.[7,8] Students should also be provided access to a standard collegiate dictionary, medical dictionary, and thesaurus for their use during clerkship rotations.

Once students have completed a written work, their preceptor should edit it using a coaching approach. Rather than simply identifying an error or unclear phrase, sentence or paragraph, suggest specific corrections or even offer completely rewritten alternative sentences in the margin of drafts under review. Writers improve when better writers edit their work. After students are provided with feedback in this way, they are better prepared to accurately and clearly articulate similar thoughts and information in the future. Therefore, editing serves two roles—to improve the writing of the moment and to improve future writing.

Preceptors may also need to assist students with particular writing challenges, such as overcoming writer's block or improving the writing of students who are not native-English speakers. A variety of writing resources are available at most colleges, and preceptors should familiarize themselves with those resources. A word of caution, however; many writing clinics are established to guide liberal arts and general education students, and their staff is often unfamiliar with technical conventions used in biomedical writing.

Finally, new preceptors working with students often find the opportunity to complete projects that are worthy of publication in peer-reviewed journals. Manuscript preparation is particularly challenging, but it can also be exceptionally rewarding for preceptors and students. Pharmacy faculty can often provide guidance, support, and assistance in that effort.

References

1. Wilkin NE. *Handbook for Pharmacy Educators: Contemporary Teaching Principles and Strategies.* Binghamptom, NY: Pharmaceutical Products Press; 2000.
2. Tindall WN, Beardsley RS, Kimberlin CL. *Communication Skills in Pharmacy Practice.* 4th ed. Philadelphia, PA: Lippincott Williams & Wilkins; 2003.
3. Hobson EH, Waite NM, Briceland LL. Writing tasks performed by doctor of pharmacy students during clerkship rotations. *Am J Health-Syst Pharm*. 2002;59:58–62.
4. Kennicutt JD, Hobson EH, Briceland LL, et al. On-the-job writing tasks of clerkship preceptors. *Am J Health-Syst Pharm*. 2002;59:63–7.
5. Pugh MB, ed. *American Medical Association Manual of Style*. 9th ed. Chicago, IL: American Medical Association; 1998.
6. Strunk W, White EB. *The Elements of Style*. 4th ed. Neeham Heights, MA: Allyn and Bacon; 2000. Available at http://www.bartleby.com/141/. Accessed May 23, 2004.
7. Hensel PR. Common student writing problems. Florida State University. Available at http://garnet.acns.fsu.edu/~phensel/problems.html#specific. Accessed May 23, 2004.
8. Lynch J. The Jack Lynch guide to grammar and style. Rutgers University. Available at http://andromeda.rutgers.edu/~jlynch/Writing/index.html. Accessed May 23, 2004.

Teach this triple truth to all: A generous heart, kind speech, and a life of service and compassion are the things which renew humanity.

Buddha

Interpersonal Skills: Warmth, Interest, Compassion

Stacy A. Taylor

Modeling Professional Relationships

As preceptors, students will look to you to gain from your wisdom and experiences in all aspects of performing your job. We generally think that experiential rotations provide an opportunity for students to begin applying their knowledge of the appropriate uses of medications, and that as preceptors, we need to serve as resources to augment and supplement this knowledge base. While this is true, our daily actions will also provide a model of how a pharmacist functions to fit into the health care world. Many students begin pharmacy school with very limited exposure to health care professionals. By observing and working alongside practicing pharmacists, students begin to develop their attitudes and abilities to interact with others. Therefore, it is important to continue to develop your skills of working with other health care professionals as well as your skills of interacting with the students you are precepting. A secondary benefit of forming strong relationships with colleagues and peers is the potential for greater career advancement and enhanced psychosocial support.[1]

Interpersonal Skills Needed for Precepting

Students who are just beginning a new rotation are often nervous or intimidated about being placed in a patient care situation in which they lack confidence and experience. The first few moments of positive interaction between students and a preceptor can quickly begin to put the students at ease. Students are more relaxed and learn better when they have a preceptor who is enthusiastic, friendly, and pleasant to be around. Students can easily perceive whether or not the preceptor is happy to have them and interested in their academic and personal needs.

As a preceptor, it is beneficial to develop professional friendships with your students and future colleagues. Students may have a variety of personal struggles outside of their professional life ranging from family illness to financial hardship. On the other hand, students may also struggle through a rotation due to lack of adequate sleep, preparation, or commitment to the rotation. When you have a good rapport with students and you know the true reason for a particular student's tardiness or failure to complete an assignment, it is easier to provide an empathetic and appropriate response. An understanding and caring preceptor can offer encouragement to students facing difficult times or can attempt to motivate wayward students. Regardless of the situation, it is difficult to meet students' academic needs without first displaying a caring and compassionate attitude toward students as individuals.

It is often difficult to maintain confidence in your own knowledge base when students seem to know all the latest information on a particular medication or disease state. This can be especially challenging for young practitioners or for seasoned practitioners who are new at precepting. However, when interacting with students it is important to convey confidence in yourself and the services you provide. Remember all of your experience and demonstrated competencies. It is not necessary for you to be an expert on all subjects in order for you to be a successful preceptor. Be a lifelong learner and take the opportunity to learn new concepts from students; it will only strengthen the bond when students realize that you are willing to listen and learn.

Skills Needed for the Development of Professional Relationships

Friendliness

We have all heard the saying "It's not always what you know, but who you know and how well you know them." Although we may not agree with the politics that surround this concept, it seems that this is how the world operates at times. For this reason it is important that you strive to develop healthy professional relationships with coworkers and members of various health care disciplines. The best way to form friendships is to be friendly, kind, and considerate. Make

◆ **Preceptor Pearls**

Take a moment to think of a pharmacist who nearly everyone enjoys being around, who has a good rapport with professional colleagues from various disciplines. Most likely, you did not think of the person who just hung up the phone on someone, is continuously grumbling under his or her breath, and is already having a bad day by 8 a.m.! Instead, the person you imagined could probably be described as someone who is kind, friendly, compassionate, empathetic, trustworthy, self-confident, optimistic, respectful of others, and maintains integrity of character. Displaying these qualities may come naturally or they may take some work, but ultimately the goal is to cultivate these skills in order to develop better relationships and have more opportunities to impact patient care.

a conscious effort to smile and interact with people at work. Develop a genuine interest in others. Ask them questions about themselves, their families, and their hobbies. In a similar manner, it is important that you be willing to share information about yourself. It is also helpful to learn some basic information about a variety of topics from sports, to politics, to current events so that you can participate in some of the most common workplace conversations. Your friendliness will make other people more comfortable coming to you with their medication-related questions or to ask your assistance on a drug-related topic that they just do not understand.

Optimism

Those people who tend to expect the best outcomes tend to be more pleasant to be around. Are you the type of person who sees the glass half empty or half full? There are good and bad points to every situation and whether you choose to focus on the good or the bad will predict what type of attitude you project and others' perceptions of you. Maintaining an optimistic confidence in the abilities of yourself and coworkers will often cause people to work even harder to live up to your expectations.

Trust

Building trust takes time, but it is a crucial skill for any pharmacist who wants to significantly impact patient care. Trust occurs when others respect your judgment and know that they can rely on you for credible information that can be directly applied without the need for questioning. In order to build trust, you must demonstrate consistency in your actions. Always be honest, reliable, and predictable.[2] This means that you show up for work and meetings on time, provide accurate responses to questions and honest opinions when asked, always follow through on pending issues, and meet deadlines. As you demonstrate your trustworthiness, other colleagues will begin to place more trust in you and your credibility will grow. Remember that trust takes a long time to build, can be destroyed quickly, and is much more difficult to regain a second time around.

Integrity

In developing integrity, it is important to first have a solid foundation of central beliefs and values by which you conduct your life. Daily decisions can then be made within the context of this value system. Trust and integrity go hand in hand; once integrity of character has been developed it is much easier to gain trust. People will come to rely on you to provide honest and consistent answers, backed up by sound reasoning and data, and that you will be accountable for your actions.

As you assume your role as a preceptor, remember the importance of developing good interpersonal skills. Students will be observing you as a role model for how a pharmacist interacts with other members of the health care world. Developing excellent interpersonal skills will also help you in precepting students, making them feel more at ease and comfortable in the learning environment.

References

1. Hitchcock MA, Bland CJ, Hekelman FD, et al. Professional Networks: The Influence of Colleagues on the Academic Success of Faculty. *Acad Med.* 1995;70:1108–16.
2. Robbins SP. *The Truth About Managing People*. Upper Saddle River, NJ: Prentice Hall; 2003.

Real education consists of drawing the best out of yourself.

Mahatma Ghandi

Teaching Skills

Diane B. Ginsburg

Many pharmacists that decide to teach students do so with little formal training in teaching and instructional design. Most pharmacists are very good at communicating clinical information, but the students they are precepting sometimes have difficulty applying this clinical information because of the manner in which the information is presented. Pharmacists are great at "data dumping." We provide information and expect it to be understood. Students can be easily overwhelmed by this as they are merely receiving information and not having the opportunity to think or apply it. Unfortunately, the pharmacist that is a great clinician may not be the best teacher and vice versa.

Teaching skills, like anything else, can be learned. Today's students respond well in an active learning environment. They need to actually try out and apply the information that is being taught. For example, a preceptor can explain the important aspects of sterile technique; however, unless the students actually compound a sterile parenteral solution, they will probably not develop the critical skills necessary to learn this technique. The majority of training students have prior to starting their experiential rotations has been in didactic lectures and simulations. For many students, rotations are the first time they have had the opportunity to apply all of this information in a real-life setting.

It is easy to understand why many preceptors do not engage in active learning. When students have a question, it is sometimes easier to just answer the question versus directing the students to research the information. The end result of this is that students probably will not remember what you told them because they have not "owned" the information. In addition, sometimes directing students to "look up the answer" can generate additional questions that must be addressed by preceptors.

There are many ways that preceptors can improve their teaching skills. Many schools offer or require specific preceptor continuing education. Frequently, these types of workshops and programs cover everything from teaching skills to assessment.

Show me someone who has done something worthwhile, and I'll show you someone who has oversome adversity.

Lou Holtz

Leadership Skills

Randy Ball

Preceptors should be recognized as leaders within their practice sites and within the profession and should help their students to recognize and understand what skills are required to become a leader. Being a leader is an active process; a preceptor cannot be a leader without being involved in the pharmacy, seeking ways to improve patient care and departmental operations.

Leadership skills required in the precepting process include leading by example, inspiring students to become actively involved, and encouraging students to achieve success. It is important for preceptors to recognize that these skills are necessary and work to strengthen these aspects. Continual development as a leader is as important for a preceptor as continual development in clinical practice or management.

Preceptors have the unique opportunity to teach students the importance of leadership within the workplace. Students may not recognize the leadership required for a pharmacist to intervene in a patient's therapy; however, the pharmacist is often the professional that is leading the process for improved patient care in these instances. By modeling this behavior, preceptors can show students in a real life situation the importance of pharmacists being leaders. Preceptors can also lead by example in dealings with students and with other health care professionals. Preceptors cannot espouse one set of behaviors as the expected norm and then exhibit a different set of behaviors. Preceptors cannot tell how important teamwork is, then talk negatively about nurses when they are not around. Preceptors cannot tell how important it is to allow pharmacists to practice clinical pharmacy, then ridicule a clinical decision another pharmacist makes. Preceptors must show students that professionalism is important. This is a key aspect of leadership for preceptors. Preceptors must set the example for professionalism for students to follow, and then they must hold students to that same level of professionalism. A preceptor who leads by example is a powerful role model for students.

Throughout a rotation, preceptors will have the opportunity to inspire students to become involved in the activities of the department and the activities of the profession. Inspiring students to become involved is a valuable way to teach rudimentary leadership skills. Engaging others in one's vision is crucial for the success of the project. Both preceptors and students must realize that great gains are seldom made alone and involving others brings the value of diverse ideas and skills to projects. Some students are easily inspired, while others test the preceptor's ability to engage. To maximize the benefit of the rotation, it is essential that preceptors can inspire students. To have this skill, preceptors must feel that their job in precepting is of utmost importance, giving them the internal desire to engage students in the rotation.

As students progress through a rotation, it is important for preceptors to look for opportunities to encourage students. Students are often trying to balance the stresses of the rotation with a job or family commitments outside of the rotation. When preceptors find ways to encourage students throughout the rotation, students will progress further and will be better able to manage the stresses of the rotation. Preceptors may share individual experiences with students and explain how to balance different aspects of life. Often students need encouragement as the rotation progresses, to balance the constructive criticism preceptors use to help students learn to apply knowledge to real life situations. Preceptors must recognize the importance of taking the time to encourage students, as well as providing feedback on their progress. This is not normally a part of a preceptor's daily routine, especially in clinical rotations. When preceptors can focus on this aspect of leadership throughout the rotation, the students' learning experience will quickly progress.

These are just a few of the leadership skills that preceptors can exhibit during the rotation period. Often preceptors are leaders within their practice sites and can use their ongoing projects as opportunities to expand student knowledge of the commitment and dedication it takes to be a leader within the profession.

Motivation is like food for the brain. You cannot get enough in one sitting. It needs continual and regular top ups.

Peter Davies

Student Expectations of a Proficient Preceptor

Kali S. Sommer

When beginning to understand the depths of student expectations of a proficient preceptor, one must first look at the big picture of where the individual student is in the course of their curriculum. Additionally, student expectations will vary due to their ability to be self-motivators. By becoming involved and engaged in this process and through evaluating student expectations, one can clearly assess student needs.

Considerations for Meeting Student Expectations

- Being an effective mentor of their development.
- Providing appropriate guidance and feedback to questions and concerns in a timely manner.
- Challenging the ability to learn in different environments.
- Fostering trust and/or collegial relationship.
- Having the ability to observe students closely versus knowing when to let go.

Students need a mentor that will be effective in their development. Precise goals and objectives should be set forth, representing an agreement between preceptors and students of the responsibilities required for successful completion of their rotation. Preceptors should also provide documentation of their current job responsibilities along with contact information, and, if possible, a work schedule. Providing pertinent information at the beginning of the rotation is an effective mechanism in teaching students where to retrieve answers to their questions on the requirements of the rotation as well as eliminating unclear expectations. Also, by providing this vision it sets students up for success.[1]

Appropriate guidance and feedback is critical so students can effectively manage areas that need improvement. Providing continuous feedback (perhaps on a weekly basis) will help relieve any anxiety that students may have. This also promotes confidence building when areas of responsibility are improved and goals and objectives are met. Types of feedback that will be helpful to students include letters of recommendation based on performance and written evaluations at the midpoint and end of rotation.

Becoming an effective pharmacist requires learning in multiple environments. Most often, patient cases do not follow the textbook approach; therefore, students expect questions from preceptors that develop their abilities to translate lectures and textbook learning to the patient. Students expect these questions to build on their drug knowledge and provide dimensions on which more clinical aspects can be applied. Also, for students to move into a "real world" position, they need to understand the process beyond clinical areas. One way to demonstrate this is to have students shadow preceptors for the course of a day so they can familiarize themselves with meetings, e-mail communication, research, and other administrative duties.

Students look up to their preceptors and enjoy learning from them. Students strive to hone as many skills as possible from their preceptors; therefore, beginning a collegial relationship and developing trust in the relationship allows students to get a level of understanding that aids in their success. For example, relationship building may include learning the students' areas of interest, and if these areas of interest are within the preceptors' scope of practice, then asking students if they would want to shadow after hours (perhaps on weekends and/or after the rotational experience is completed). Also, building relationships between preceptors and students helps students understand why preceptors do things a certain way and demonstrate levels of prioritizing. This type of relationship building fosters success skills beyond the clinical learning environment. It also allows preceptors to better understand students and, therefore, better assess their situational learning.

Finally, student ability to become skillful pharmacists depends on the preceptor's ability to know when to give further guidance and when to let go. It is imperative to their success that students develop in their roles as pharmacists, become efficient in the process, and are able to go the direction alone.

Reference

1. Collins JC, Porras JI. *Built to Last: Successful Habits of Visionary Companies*. New York: HarperCollins Publishers; 1997.

The happiest life is that which constantly exercises and educates what is best in us.

Philip G. Hamerton

Why Being a Preceptor is an Important Aspect of Pharmacy Practice

Randy Ball

The practice of pharmacy is a proud profession with a rich history and many varied practice settings. The future of pharmacy will be determined by recent and future graduates. These graduates rely heavily on experiential rotations for developing their foundation in pharmacy practice today and what it can be in the future.

Each practice setting has unique experiences that can be utilized to teach students how to practice pharmacy in a real world environment. Through experiential rotations, students learn how to apply the knowledge they have acquired through their pharmacy school coursework. Students also learn how to be professionals and how to interact with other health care practitioners. Precepted experiential rotations provide students with the opportunity to learn how to provide pharmaceutical care within various practice settings, while under the guidance of a skilled practitioner.

In addition to the value precepting has for the students, precepting rotations also provides value to the practice site. Hosting students on experiential rotations provides the site with an infusion of intelligent practitioners who help to keep the pharmacy knowledge base sharpened. Journal clubs and formal presentations provide pharmacy staff, both professional and technical, with up-to-date pharmacy information. Students who have completed interesting rotations also serve as positive advertising for the pharmacy among their classmates as they begin to seek employment after graduation.

In addition to the benefit to students and training sites, precepting is also professionally rewarding for preceptors. They have the opportunity to influence future practitioners and, in doing so, can influence the future of the profession for many years to come. Precepting also helps preceptors to be sharpened, as they reinforce their own knowledge and expand their own horizons through student interactions. As preceptors answer questions and explain pharmacy practice, they gain an even deeper understanding of their own practice. Routine daily tasks that are frequently done without much thought become fresh again as they are explained to students. Taking time to befriend students also creates a unique professional bond that can last beyond the rotation period. It is not uncommon for former students to maintain contact with their preceptors who helped to shape their professional perspective.

Overall, precepting experiential rotations is one of the most important aspects of pharmacy practice when done correctly. When the time and resources are devoted to making the rotation a top notch experience, the students, the preceptor, and the site all benefit. Ultimately, patient care is improved, and this is the reason we practice pharmacy.

Originality is the essence of truc scholarship. Creativity is the soul of the true scholar.

Benjamin Nnamdi Azikiwe

New Ideas for Seasoned Preceptors

Kevin Purcell

Seasoned preceptors often like to experiment with implementing new ideas and concepts into their internship programs. This provides some new challenges and excitement for preceptors as well as some new learning opportunities for students. Preceptors can either formulate unique and innovative ideas that are true revolutionary advances in student education, or they can simply add a different spin to the ideas and practices of others.

Preceptors could require students to assemble a competency portfolio during the internship that documents their competency in the desired areas. This would be consistent with the movement in health care to better assess the competency of students, residents, and practitioners with the ultimate goal of improving patient safety and outcomes (clinical, economic, and humanistic). Competency is difficult to assess because it is composed of multiple domains including knowledge, skills, abilities, values, attitudes, beliefs, and behaviors. No single evaluation method (e.g., examinations, assignments, direct observation, etc.) can be used to accurately and appropriately assess competency in all of these areas. Competency assessment really requires the use of a variety of methods and instruments.

One way to demonstrate competency is through use of a comprehensive competency portfolio, which may have some similarity to a diary (e.g., reflective writing on feelings and experiences) and to a promotion and/or tenure dossier of a faculty member (e.g., demonstration of activity and achievement in certain areas including practice, teaching, research, and service). Of course, the first step is to define the desired areas of competency for students. Preceptors should check with their respective academic programs to determine if this requirement exists and then incorporate it into their experiential program. The pharmacy schools with which preceptors are affiliated may have already done this. If not, preceptors can take the lead and develop a set of competencies that they expect students to have after completion of their internship. The Accreditation Council for Graduate Medical Education requires that all medical and surgical residency programs implement methods to assess and document competency of their graduates in the following six areas by June 2006: patient care, medical knowledge, practice-based learning and improvement, interpersonal and communication skills, professionalism, and systems-based practice.[1] Also, the American Association of Colleges of Pharmacy has developed a set of educational outcomes (Appendix I).[2] A list of some example pharmacy practice competencies that could be further defined by preceptors and used to assess students is provided in Table 4.2. Students can demonstrate how each competency has been attained through a variety of documents in a competency portfolio as well as by doing some self-assessment and reflective writing related to each competency. Each competency could have its own section in a three-ring binder, and the same binder could probably contain the internship manual (the internship syllabus and other useful information) and the competency portfolio materials. Some potential contents that could be included in a competency portfolio are listed in Table 4.3.

Preceptors could find ways to apply art, music, poetry, and literature to pharmacy practice and student education in order to help students develop their humanistic qualities and broaden their cultural education. Some art, music, poetry, and literature can portray an expression of the artist's/author's feelings and experiences with disease, the health care system, and society. Using art, music, poetry, and literature for teaching purposes can help students see illness and treatment from their patients' perspectives and comprehend their patients' suffering so that they can accompany them through illnesses with empathy, respect, and effective care. Studying and trying to interpret art, music, poetry, and literature also can help sharpen observational skills (seeing what is present and not present) and listening skills (hearing what patients are really saying). Although it can be difficult to detect subtle meaning in pictures and phrases, it can be just as difficult to understand the significance of the tone of a patient's words, the inflection of his/her voice, and his/her facial expressions and body language.

There are multiple ways to incorporate the visual or performing arts as well as literature and poetry into an internship, and preceptors are only limited by their own creativity and artistic ability. Critically evaluating artwork, especially paintings and photographs of people, can enhance and hone observational skills.[3] A trip to a local art museum could be incorporated into the internship and occur on the weekend. Alternatively, art books or slides could be used at the practice site, but some of the culturally enhancing atmosphere may be lost. The most powerful aspect of physical examination is observation. One can obtain a lot of relevant medical information just from carefully observing someone, describing what is seen, and interpreting the findings. Observing, describing, and interpreting artwork can help develop these skills. Revealing the history of the artwork and what the artists meant to convey can complete the exercise. Also, patients have written many books and poems about coping with their diseases. Students could be required to read some selected books and poems to better understand things from patients' perspectives. Seeing things through patients' eyes may make students appreciate the strength of a holistic model of patient care that addresses the mind, body, and spirit and considers all the various factors that affect health and well-being (see Figure 4-2).[4,5] Often health care professionals focus only on treating patients' diseases (the physical aspect) but ignore psychological, spiritual, socioeconomic, cultural, and environmental factors that affect their patients' health care outcomes. Finally,

Table 4.2 • *Example Pharmacy Practice Competencies*

- *Leadership and teamwork*
- *Professionalism*
- *Interpersonal and communication/listening skills*
- *Cultural awareness/sensitivity*
- *Pharmaceutical and medical knowledge*
- *Individual and population-based patient care*
- *Pharmacy operations, clinical services, and practice management*
- *Computers and technology*
- *Evidence and systems-based practice, management, and continuous quality improvement*
- *Personal and professional growth and development*

Table 4.3 • *Potential Contents in a Competency Portfolio*

- *De-identified patient care plans*
- *Case studies or problem sets*
- *Literature search results*
- *Formulary monographs*
- *Drug use evaluations*
- *Patient information leaflets*
- *Term papers*
- *Research or process improvement projects*
- *Publications (case reports, review articles, studies, commentaries, etc.) and posters*
- *Presentation handouts (inservices, etc.)*
- *Certifications*
- *Patient care log (number of patients seen with each condition)*
- *Intervention log (number and type of interventions made)*
- *Procedure log (number and type of clinical and operational procedures performed)*
- *Meeting attendance log (e.g., hospital, professional society, community support group)*
- *Reading log (books, chapters, articles, etc.)*
- *Professional service activities*
- *Community service activities*
- *Self-assessment exercises (Myers-Briggs personality test, Haygroup emotional intelligence inventory, Kouzes and Posner leadership skills inventory, etc.)*
- *Letters of appreciation from patients, physicians, and other health care professionals*
- *Awards*
- *Individual development plan*
- *Reflective writing (what students have learned and how they have grown and developed through certain experiences)*

reading essays, poems, and books written by pharmacists or other practitioners may also help students understand what it means to be a pharmacist and a health care professional.

Preceptors can create a practice model for students with defined duties and responsibilities that are important functions and aspects of patient care and pharmacy operations. Often students do not have clearly defined roles at practice sites, and they are not well integrated into the patient care process or the pharmacy operations. Of course, it is hard for preceptors to essentially create an unsalaried job position and description for students if they do not have a constant supply of students. Student intern positions with important duties and responsibilities would have to be filled year-round to provide consistency and continuity of services, especially if the students are integrated into a patient care unit and team in a hospital. Once expectations of other health care professionals have been built and met by students providing them support for patient care services, there cannot be lapses in coverage. The practice site will need to always have a student in that position. This will require a strong partnership with one or more pharmacy schools in order to meet the site's demand for students.

For example, under the supervision of a pharmacist preceptor, students can be decentralized to a patient care unit or team in a hospital and provide a spectrum of pharmacy services. Students could be responsible for a number of functions including taking initial medication histories; conducting daily drug regimen reviews; answering drug information questions; performing therapeutic drug monitoring services; writing patient care plans and daily progress notes; reviewing discharge medications; counseling patients; and providing inservices to the medical, nursing, and allied health staff. Students also could act as liaisons for the pharmacy department and help nurses on the patient care units and centralized staff pharmacists troubleshoot problems with the medication use system (prescribing, dispensing, administration, and monitoring). Students can be provided a pager so that the unit, team, and preceptor can always reach them.

Although the above example is for creating a student practice model in an inpatient unit, student practice models related to patient care services or pharmacy operations and management could be developed in many other pharmacy practice settings. Also, when at all possible, preceptors should get senior students involved in more advanced practice activities and involve other professionals (e.g., physicians, nurses, dietitians, respiratory therapists, business manager) in their internships as copreceptors to provide specific education and experiences. Advanced practice activities can include disease screenings; patient assessment (physical examination, laboratory test interpretation, etc.); medication administration; drug therapy and disease management; patient counseling

Figure 4-2 • Holistic Model for Patient Care

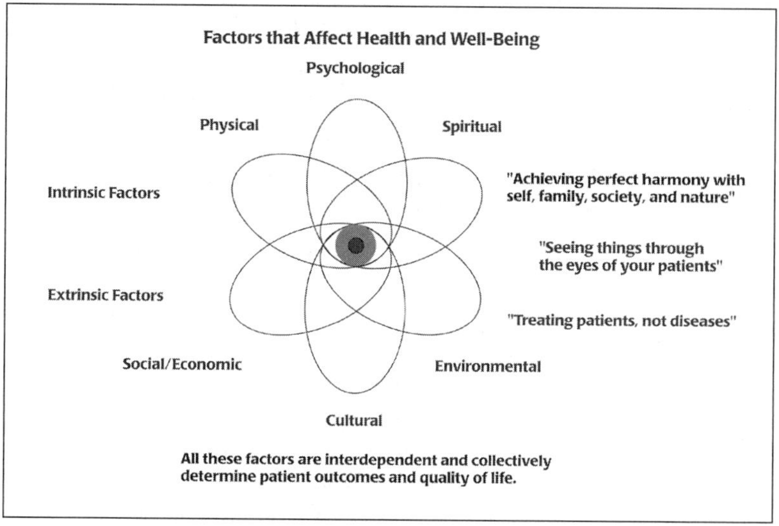

on health promotion/disease prevention and on their diseases and medications; and practice and financial management. Additionally, teaching by students could be incorporated into the internship in a couple of ways such as providing inservices to health care professions and educating support groups about drug therapy and disease management. Teaching really forces one to fully understand the material.

Preceptors can encourage students to present and publish their work on projects or their thoughts on issues. Presenting and publishing are excellent educational activities, and they also bring recognition. There are multiple places for students to present (e.g., local, state, and national pharmacy society meetings, community organization meetings) or publish (e.g., employer or professional society newsletters, local and national newspapers, state and national pharmacy society journals) their work or thoughts. Often students are required to complete a project (research, process improvement, community service, etc.) or an assignment (formulary monograph, therapeutic review, etc.) that could be presented or published in a variety of forums. Also, sometimes students see patients with significant clinical findings that are either unusual or new and not previously reported, which could be written up as a brief case report. Thoughts on issues can be submitted as viewpoints, opinions, commentaries, or letters to the editor to many newsletters, newspapers, and journals. Sometimes background research done for finding answers to patient care problems, developing policies and procedures, or conducting formulary evaluations can be written up as a review article for a newsletter or journal. Overall, writing articles of any type can reinforce learning, enhance written communication skills, and stimulate one to clarify his/her beliefs and positions.

Preceptors can also require students to participate in professional society and community service activities. Preceptors are often involved in professional societies and community service organizations but sometimes fail to get students involved, especially since the meetings tend to be in the evenings and the activities are usually on the weekends. However, preceptors need to take students with them to these functions. Participation in professional societies and community service organizations is a critical element of the professionalization process and provides one of the best opportunities for leadership development. Also, preceptors do not need to give students compensatory time off during the workweek for attending evening and weekend professional society and community service activities. Preceptors do not get compensatory time off from work for doing this, so students do not either. This is part of the students' learning about the life of a pharmacist who is dedicated to public service, the advancement of pharmacy practice and patient care, and lifelong learning. Some colleges of pharmacy recognize attendance of outside professional organizational meetings as "Special Activity Hours" and give credit for these during the rotation.

Preceptors must keep in mind that more than anything else students want to be able to spend quality time talking with and learning from them. Often because of the hectic nature of many practice environments, preceptors are not able to spare much time during the workday to do this. One way to accommodate this desire and need of students for their preceptors' time is to set aside time outside of the workday. For example, preceptors could have a cup of coffee or breakfast with students every Friday morning before work. The topics for discussion could be left up to the students since this is their special time with their preceptors. Topics could encompass everything from deciding on an initial career pathway and getting a job to discussing how to proactively address issues facing the profession though advocacy and leadership.

These are just a few of an infinite number of ideas and concepts that can be used to add value to an internship program and make the educational process more meaningful and fulfilling to both preceptors and students. The important thing is for preceptors to always find things to do that keep them challenged, excited, and energized about precepting students. Experimenting with ways to add new dimensions to internships or to completely reinvent internships can be therapeutic for preceptors and create new and better learning opportunities for students.

References

1. Accreditation Council for Graduate Medical Education. Outcome Project. Available at: http://www.acgme.org/outcome/comp/compFull.asp.
2. American Association of Colleges of Pharmacy. CAPE outcomes. Available at: http://www.aacp.org.
3. Bardes CL, Gillers D, Herman A. Learning to look: developing clinical observational skills at an art museum. *Med Educ.* 2001;35:1157–61.
4. Purcell K. Pharmacy leadership survey: developing pharmacy leaders. In press at the *Texas Society of Health-System Pharmacists Journal.*
5. Purcell K. Learning the skills and knowledge necessary to provide patient care. Texas Society of Health-System Pharmacists Newsletter. June 1996;25(4):8–9.

Time is the most precious element of human existence. The successful person knows how to put energy into time and how to draw success from time.

Denis Waitley

How to Be an Effective Preceptor While Meeting Your Employment Requirements: Integrating Pharmacy Students into Your Practice

Lourdes M. Cuéllar

Objectives

- Create ways to prepare for student arrival and integration into your practice setting.
- Assess student experience and readiness to learn.
- Create activities that provide students with the opportunity to meet all learning objectives while meeting work requirements.
- Develop methods for evaluating student performance.
- Understand the importance of developing professional relationships.
- Improve interpersonal skills between preceptor and students.
- Foster skills needed for the development of professional relationships.

Pharmacy education in most practice settings is characterized in part by balancing educational effectiveness, while simultaneously trying to provide optimal patient care. As practitioners we are all juggling multiple things while teaching and supervising students. Time constraints and the multiple pressures and deadlines are all factors that today's practitioners face. The constraints associated by high census, high volume, high patient acuity, clarifying prescriptions or medication orders, dealing with insurance problems, and staffing shortages only serve to escalate the intensity of dealing with these two important aspects of being an effective preceptor. There are educationally sound methods that incorporate time-management, organizational skills, and effective planning to assist preceptors in integrating pharmacy student education and meeting employment requirements.

Preparing for the Students' Arrival

Be prepared when students arrive at your facility or practice setting. Students appreciate structure, and it provides them with the opportunity not only to meet all learning objectives but also to be trained and participate in services and activities that are unique to your practice setting. As the preceptor you will be able to teach in a more productive manner and allow the students to have effective patient encounters with appropriate education, guidance, and supervision.

Develop a Training Manual

Begin by developing a training manual specific to your facility and experiential rotation(s). This demonstrates to the students your commitment to their education and training. Be creative when developing your manual. Begin with a welcome letter or memo. In the manual, be sure to include not only information about the pharmacy and the experiential rotation, but also information about your practice site, institution, or facility. Do not forget to include a map of your facility, especially if it is a large teaching or community hospital. Tell the story of your institution. Include an organizational map of the hospital or practice site and your department. Insert a copy of your job description. Students who have never worked in a pharmacy or seen a pharmacist in clinical practice are often surprised at the extent of duties and responsibilities and creative practice structure of pharmacists in today's health-system environments.

Prepare a Comprehensive Orientation Checklist.

Orienting the students to the training site is a well-recognized strategy for creating a positive learning experience and communicating goals, objectives, and minimal competencies for the experiential training rotation.

Orientation should include the following:

- Goals, objectives, and minimal competency requirements of the rotation.
- Rotation hours and attendance policy.
- Regulatory compliance standards relating to your State Board of Pharmacy.
- Tour of your facility and department.
- Review of required reading for the rotation.

- Terms and definitions for students completing a rotation in an unfamiliar practice setting.
- A trip to Human Resources to obtain an identification badge and complete facility orientation requirements.
- Introduction to all members of the department and a brief explanation of their duties.
- Introduction to key members of the medical, nursing, and other health professional staff (or store or office manager) that they will be working with on a day-to-day basis.
- A review of facility's policies and procedures.
- Introduction to your Pharmacy Information System.
- Introduction or review of your facility-specific medical record system.
- Review of all pertinent medication use policies (e.g., standard administration times, approved abbreviations, and substitution guidelines).
- Publications, journals, and other reference materials available to students.
- Evaluation instruments, timing and methods, exams and grading policy.

You will need to devote a significant amount of time the first week of the rotation to set expectations and ground rules. By ensuring that students have a full understanding of your expectations, there is less chance for misinterpretation or confusion later. This also makes for an easier transition to empower students to take on projects and be more independent as they move throughout the remaining weeks of the rotation (with ongoing supervision and follow-up from the preceptor).

Develop a Schedule for the Students

Build preceptor teaching time and also time for the students to reflect on their patient encounters. Be sure to include midterm and final exam dates, site-specific and school events and holidays, and assignment due dates (e.g., case presentations, journal club, patient care plan, build in a project where the patients are sure to benefit and students experiences success). Do not forget to communicate your expectations to students. Be specific.

Capitalize on your practice site and your strengths as a preceptor when developing student schedules. Assign special projects and presentations that will

◆ **PRECEPTOR PEARLS**

Develop an Institution-Specific Experiential Training Manual

- General orientation checklist
- Welcome memo or letter
- Map of hospital or practice site and important contacts or department listings
- Goals of your program
- Job description
- Background reading material—medical services or special patient populations served
- Sample formats for patient case presentations, SOAP and consult notes, journal club presentations, and intervention reports
- Schedule (include assignment due dates)
- Have a working lunch with students early on in the rotation and establish your relationship as a teacher, mentor, and soon-to-be peer

benefit both the site and students. Include patient education, literature searches, physician case conferences, morbidity and mortality rounds, pharmacy and therapeutics or formulary meetings, and grand rounds as part of their experiential training. As you review the schedule with students, be sure to allow them to ask questions and take time to explain to them how all the activities impact patient care.

Allow for student individuality and creativity. Make provisions in the schedule to allow for activities that meet specific student needs and desires. Assess their strengths and weaknesses and allow enough flexibility to meet their educational needs and interests. If you develop a project on some of their interests, they will be more motivated to perform those activities that are less interesting as well. Be flexible and try out new concepts or ideas. Most importantly, identify opportunities for student involvement when considering any and all of your planned activities.

Assess Students' Prior Experience and Readiness to Learn

Familiarize yourself with students' prior rotations, experiences, and their professional goals. Assess the students' areas of interest. Determine their short and long-term goals on day one of the rotation. Let them know that their schedule is flexible enough to allow for their involvement and input into planning their daily activities. Assess their readiness and motivation to learn. Ascertain if they have previous experience working as a pharmacy technician. For example, students may have prior experience working as an IV technician in a health-system setting. You may choose to perform a validation of their skills and then take the time normally assigned to that activity and change it to an area of particular interest to the students or on a special project or assignment.

Students generally progress through predictable stages of learning development. It is critical to the success of the rotation that preceptors take time on the first days of the rotation to ascertain each student individually. This exercise should not only determine students' basic pharmacological competency and core clinical skills, but also verbal and written communication skills, problem solving skills, and ability to perform multiple tasks and handle complex patients. As a preceptor you should be able to rapidly identify student strengths and needs relative to meeting all the learning objectives of your rotation. Have a plan, but be flexible in adjusting to meet student needs and abilities.

Set Clear Expectations

The first meeting with your students sets the tone for the entire training encounter. Ensure that students understand and accept that both of you must work together throughout the rotation to assure quality patient care as well as quality education and training.

To have a successful experiential rotation, it is absolutely vital that the preceptor establishes standards. Be specific when you communicate your expectations to students. Offer students ideas as you mutually establish specific goals for their rotation. Give them creative challenges; promote their strengths. By linking the students' performance to those standards, the preceptor creates a benchmark for achievement. The ultimate goal is to transition from a teacher/student learner relationship to clinical supervisor/responsible performer (clinician) relationship. Students should be able to demonstrate their problem-solving skills and integrate their didactic knowledge and clinical training to real daily situations. There should be a good balance between education and service.

A good preceptor should be able to relate to students how all their activities

◆ **PRECEPTOR PEARLS**

- Set the bar high and hold students to those standards.
- Link rewards and appreciation when students meet designated standards of excellence.
- Coach students to exceed their current capabilities.
- Provide an opportunity for a scholarly activity at the state or national level when possible.
- Incorporate communication skill activities when possible. A practitioner with good clinical skills cannot apply them without good communication skills.
- Ensure interactions with other providers as well as with patients.
- Demonstrate enthusiasm and the ability to stimulate students.
- Lead by example; practice what you preach.
- Demonstrate personal clinical competence.
- Practice regular clinical supervision; demonstrate interest in the students.
- Be a caring teacher.

impact patient care. Provide guidance, answer questions, explain answers, and assist students in developing self-confidence and self-esteem. An exemplary preceptor demonstrates a *can do* attitude and is dedicated to helping students achieve their full potential.

Most experiential training sites afford students the opportunity to work and train with a number of other professionals besides the primary preceptor. Choose professionals that are motivated and committed to student education. The pharmacist team of preceptors can teach students a number of critical skills that are not necessarily related to the science of pharmacy but rather the human side of our profession. Students will also be able to observe different approaches taken by the various health care professionals. Some of these critical skills include ethics, teamwork, leadership skills, empathy and compassion, and communication, as well as the technical and cognitive abilities of being a pharmacist. Introduce diverse activities that provide students with the opportunity to meet all learning objectives while meeting work requirements.

In order to be able to simultaneously provide a successful educational experience and ensure clinical effectiveness, the preceptor must be organized and identify strategies for providing educational opportunities. Orienting students to patient encounters is an effective strategy for creating a good learning environment and providing effective direct patient care. Learn to present a one to two minute patient-specific orientation. This will help students obtain a conceptual framework that will help them to efficiently interpret vital patient information. For example, the preceptor should review the patient's medical background, explain to students what symptoms or conditions to focus on, and establish guidelines for interventions, monitoring, or a patient care plan. Another example would be going over with students the importance of calling a physician if unclear about a prescription or the steps to take if they come across a drug interaction. During each patient-specific encounter, the preceptor should alert students to any potentially coexisting problems or additional medical conditions in the patient's history.

> **◆ PRECEPTOR PEARLS**
>
> Introduce activities that
> - promote active student participation.
> - emphasize applied problem solving.
> - demonstrate skillful interaction with patients and other members of the health care team.
> - place emphasis on evidence-based literature/decision making.
> - demonstrate by example multiple skills utilizing daily experiences and interactions.
> - capitalize on site and preceptor strengths.
> - meet the goals, objectives, and minimal competencies set by the school.

The patient case presentation offers both the preceptor and students an optimal opportunity for teaching and learning. Teaching with the patient allows the preceptor to observe students' performance and provide immediate feedback. The preceptor should verbally identify what students did well, and then ascertain problem areas and suggest steps students might take to correct them. Do not dictate the solution, even if it seems obvious.

The following are some examples of effective opportunities to teach in a productive manner:

- Patient education and counseling
- Pharmacotherapy, nutrition, and pharmacokinetic consults
- Literature searches
- Physician case conference or grand rounds presentations
- Performance enhancement activities such as evaluation of regulatory compliance
- MUE/DUE criteria development, data collection, queries, and compilation of results
- Provide for interdisciplinary training (e.g., shadowing a nurse, dietician, or respiratory therapist for a set number of hours)
- Technician activities
- Departmental budget preparation and review process
- Policies and procedures development or revisions and updates to staff
- Patient case presentation
- Presentation for Pharmacy & Therapeutics Committee
- Journal Club
- Drug information questions
- Inservices for nurses, pharmacists, medical residents, and other disciplines
- Special projects, presentations, or experiences

Remember that students should be active participants. Care must be taken not to make any pertinent learning activities a mere "shadowing" experience. Students should know the reason or rationale for the activity or project.

Promote self-directed learning. At the end of the day ask "What did you learn today?" or "What medical problem or condition would you like to learn more about?" or "What was the most important thing you learned today?" Link self-directed learning to a recently observed patient problem or departmental process or procedure. Self-directed learning can also include research, literature review, or selected reading about a disease or condition that is prevalent in the patient population you serve. Self-directed learning should apply the

> ◆ **Preceptor Pearls**
> **Effective Teaching toward Competency**
> - Demonstrate by role modeling
> - Coach and observe practice performance
> - Provide clinical supervision
> - Give constructive feedback
> - Recognize achievements

students' didactic knowledge to real life patient encounters or experiences.

A very effective teaching tactic is service-based education. There are two specific means of utilizing this teaching strategy. The first is by identifying tasks that are routinely performed by nonlicensed staff in your department or other health care providers. The second is community service-based education.

Within the department allow students to spend some time with the support staff. Have them perform duties such as triaging patient or nursing phone calls, assisting at the service window, calling insurance companies, retrieving charts, repackaging medications, calling physicians to clarify orders, and assisting in the ordering and inventory process. This helps students comprehend and appreciate how each employee is a valuable member of the pharmacy team. It is also important for students to learn how these functions are critical to the operations of the department.

It is imperative that students learn the value of community service education as part of their experiential training. Start by inviting them to go with you to one of your local pharmacy organizations' continuing education programs. Teach them the value of fellowship and networking with colleagues within your community.

If you are actively involved in any volunteer community activities, such as local health fairs, providing health care to the homeless, serving food at local shelters, or volunteering at a clinic for indigent families, invite the students to go with you. Give them specific goals such as learning about the following:

- The role of community agencies, nursing homes, hospices, and public agencies, programs, and clinics.
- Professionalism and community spirit and advocacy.
- How community health services are funded.

- How to practice preventative medicine.
- The social, economic, and ethical aspects of health care.

Give the students observation questions or assignments. Help them to see the "big picture" of health care as well as the specifics of patient care. For example:

- What services are provided to the patient?
- List the disciplines and their roles within the clinic or facility.
- How do pharmacists interact with this site?
- Name some ways in which literacy is a public health issue.
- Identify common reasons why a physician orders home health or hospice care.
- List physical findings consistent with domestic violence or abuse.
- Describe the role of the hospital chaplain.
- Briefly define the care rendered at a skilled nursing facility and the role of the pharmacist.

Develop a community service site directory and let students choose where they would like to visit. Examples of places that are good learning environments for students include the following:

- Adult or Child Protective Services
- City/county clinics or emergency room
- Hospital social work department
- Child development in a pediatric unit
- Local substance abuse program
- Nursing home care unit
- Visiting nurse association
- Hospital chaplaincy
- Local AIDS clinic

The most useful activity after community service education is reflection. Focus on a teaching point. Were the patient concerns addressed effectively? The preceptor should provide meaningful feedback and ask if the expectations were realistic and reasonable for the students. The goal is to help students realize that the contributions they can make go beyond the work place environment. The professional rewards of the service-oriented teaching are great, and students recognize the value of intrinsic rewards such as personal and professional growth and development.

Provide Ongoing Feedback

Spend time with the students having lunch in the cafeteria. Ask questions about their learning experience. Provide frequent assessment; informal assessment should be ongoing throughout the rotation. In your informal conversations discuss issues such as lifetime learning habits, the role of residency training, balancing career and family goals, applying for a job, and interview skills.

> ◆ **PRECEPTOR PEARLS**
>
> Take them out to lunch on their last day of rotation; celebrate with the students as they complete their rotation. Think of rewards such as lunch with the "team," or give them a textbook, leadership book, or other book on a topic you have been discussing. Ask students for feedback on how you can be a better preceptor or in what ways that the experiential rotation could be improved.

Sit down with students at least once a week to provide formal feedback and assessment. Review the progress that they have made and give them the opportunity to come up with ways to improve areas that need to be strengthened. Be candid. Provide honest and constructive feedback. Listen carefully to students when you ask them for their self-assessment.

Acknowledge student contributions. Do so in front of other members of the health care team or during a departmental staff meeting. This will go a long way in helping build self-esteem. Help them promote their strengths and teach them to assume broader responsibilities in meeting their educational goals.

Do not forget to bring in some real life experiences. Tell them about your preceptors and mentors and the influence they had on your life. As much as possible, be accessible and approachable to the students. Develop a mentor-protégé relationship if possible.

Secrets of Success

Both the preceptor and the students must be committed to providing patient care and to pharmacy education. The preceptor must consistently demonstrate competency and professionalism and have a passion for education, service, and excellence. Consistency and standardization are essential for effective teaching and integrating pharmacy students into your practice. Effective planning, comprehensive student orientation, setting clear expectations, introducing diverse learning experiences, and ongoing constructive feedback are integral to the students' successful learning experience.

The main part of intellectual education is not the acquisition of facts but learning how to make facts live.

Oliver Wendell Holmes

How to Become a Preceptor—Summary of Common School of Pharmacy Requirements and States with Unique Requirements

Vikki Jill Polk, Diane B. Ginsburg

There are many requirements for individual practitioners to become involved in teaching in the experiential component of the curriculum. A summary of the requirements for preceptors by academic institution is listed in Table 4.4 (see next page).

Licensure

Licensure is not a component in Table 4.4 because most schools and colleges of pharmacy require that a licensed pharmacist supervise students. If a school is listed with no additional information or an asterisk, then that school only requires supervision by a licensed pharmacist. Specific institutions do require that if the state's board or regulatory agent licenses or registers preceptors, the pharmacist must be in compliance with the state's procedures before precepting students. However, some institutions will allow preceptors to be individuals with appropriate professional degrees and/or experience.

Specific Requirements

Some schools and colleges have specific requirements, credentials, or qualifications that must be met in order for a preceptor to supervise students. This is an area that has a great deal of variance among the institutions. Requirements can range from a strong desire to teach students to specifically being involved in professional organizations. The institutions listed having specific requirements provide information to pharmacists wanting to precept students. The following

Table 4.4 • *School of Pharmacy Requirements*

Pharmacy College/ School	Specific Requirements	Length of Practice	Documents	Approval	Training	Legal Standing
Harrison–Auburn University	*Yes*		*Yes*		*Yes*	*Yes*
McWhorter–Samford University	*Yes*					
Glendale Midwestern University			*Yes*	*Yes*		
The University of Arizona	*Yes*		*Yes*	*Yes*		
University of Arkansas for Medical Science	*Yes*		*Yes*	*Yes*		
University of California, San Francisco/San Diego	*Yes*		*Yes*			
*University of the Pacific, Thomas J. Long**		*2 semesters***	*Yes*	*Yes*		*Yes*
University of Southern California	*Yes*		*Yes*		*Yes*	
Western University of Health Sciences	*Yes*		*Yes*	*Yes*		
University of Colorado, Health Sciences Center	*Yes*					
University of Connecticut	*Yes*	*1 y*		*Yes*	*Yes*	
Howard University	*Yes*	*2 y*		*Yes*		
Florida Agriculture and Mechanical University						
*Nova Southeastern University**	*Yes*		*Yes*	*Yes*		
Palm Beach Atlantic University	*Yes*	*2 y*		*Yes*	*Yes*	
*University of Florida**	*Yes*		*Yes*	*Yes*		
Mercer University	*Yes*	*1 y*				*Yes*
*The University of Georgia**	*Yes*	*1 y*	*Yes*		*Yes*	
Idaho State University	*Yes*					
Midwestern University		*6 mo***	*Yes*	*Yes*	*Yes*	
University of Illinois at Chicago	*Yes*		*Yes*	*Yes*		
Butler University		*2 y***	*Yes*			
Purdue University	*Yes*					*Yes*
Drake University	*Yes*	*1 y*	*Yes*	*Yes*		*Yes*
The University of Iowa	*Yes*					*Yes*
University of Kansas		*2 y*				*Yes*
The University of Kentucky	*Yes*		*Yes*	*Yes*		*Yes*
The University of Louisiana at Monroe	*Yes*		*Yes*		*Yes*	*Yes*
*Xavier University of Louisiana**	*Yes*	*2 y*				
*University of Maryland**	*Yes*		*Yes*			

Table 4.4 • *School of Pharmacy Requirements (continued)*

Pharmacy College/ School	Specific Requirements	Length of Practice	Documents	Approval	Training	Legal Standing
Massachusetts–Boston	*Yes*	*1 y*			*Yes*	*Yes*
Massachusetts–Worcester						
Northeastern University–Bouve College						
Ferris State University				*Yes*		
*The University of Michigan**	*Yes*		*Yes*	*Yes*	*Yes*	
Wayne State University–Eugene Applebaum	*Yes*	*1 y*		*Yes*		
University of Minnesota and Duluth Branch			*Yes*	*Yes*		
The University of Mississippi	*Yes*	*3 y*	*Yes*	*Yes*	*Yes*	*Yes*
St. Louis College of Pharmacy	*Yes*		*Yes*	*Yes*	*Yes*	
*University of Missouri–Kansas City**						
The University of Montana	*Yes*	*2 y*				
Creighton University			*Yes*	*Yes*		
University of Nebraska	*Yes*	*1 y*			*Yes*	*Yes*
Nevada College of Pharmacy	*Yes*		*Yes*		*Yes*	
Rutgers, Ernest Mario						
The University of New Mexico		*1 y*	*Yes*	*Yes*		
Arnold and Marie Schwartz	*Yes*					
St. John's University						
University of Buffalo	*Yes*	*1 y*	*Yes*	*Yes*		*Yes*
Union University, Albany	*Yes*					
Campbell University	*Yes*					*Yes*
University of North Carolina	*Yes*			*Yes*	*Yes*	
North Dakota State University					*Yes*	
Ohio Northern University	*Yes*		*Yes*		*Yes*	
The Ohio State University	*Yes*		*Yes*		*Yes*	
University of Cincinnati–Medical Center	*Yes*	*1 y*	*Yes*	*Yes*	*Yes*	*Yes*
The University of Toledo	*Yes*				*Yes*	
*Southwestern Oklahoma State University**	*Yes*					
University of Oklahoma	*Yes*		*Yes*	*Yes*		*Yes*
Oregon State University	*Yes*					
Duquesne University						
*Lake Erie College of Osteopathic Medicine**						

Table 4.4 • *School of Pharmacy Requirements (continued)*

Pharmacy College/ School	Specific Requirements	Length of Practice	Documents	Approval	Training	Legal Standing
University of Sciences in Philadelphia	*Yes*		*Yes*	*Yes*		
Temple University			*Yes*	*Yes*		*Yes*
University of Pittsburgh	*Yes*			*Yes*	*Yes*	
*Wilkes University**	*Yes*	*3 y*		*Yes*		*Yes*
University of Rhode Island			*Yes*	*Yes*		
Medical University of South Carolina	*Yes*	*1 y*	*Yes*			
*University of South Carolina**		*2 y*	*Yes*			
South Dakota State University	*Yes*		*Yes*		*Yes*	
University of Tennessee			*Yes*	*Yes*		
Texas Southern University	*Yes*	*1 y*	*Yes*	*Yes*	*Yes*	*Yes*
Texas Tech University			*Yes*	*Yes*		
The University of Houston	*Yes*	*1 y*		*Yes*		*Yes*
The University of Texas at Austin	*Yes*	*1 y*	*Yes*	*Yes*	*Yes*	
University of Utah		*1 y ***	*Yes*	*Yes*	*Yes*	
Hampton University	*Yes*	*2 y*	*Yes*		*Yes*	*Yes*
Shenandoah University, Bernard J. Dunn	*Yes*		*Yes*	*Yes*		
Virginia Commonwealth University	*Yes*			*Yes*		
University of Washington	*Yes*					
Washington State University	*Yes*	*1 y*	*Yes*	*Yes*	*Yes*	
West Virginia University			*Yes*	*Yes*	*Yes*	
University of Wisconsin, Madison	*Yes*	*1 y*	*Yes*	*Yes*	*Yes*	
University of Wyoming		*2 y*		*Yes*		*Yes*

***Require licensed/registered preceptors**: Auburn University, the University of Arkansas for Medical Science, the University of Colorado Health Sciences Center (only if participating in traditional clerkships), the University of Kentucky (if such process is in place for the professional), the University of Louisiana at Monroe, Xavier University, Ferris State University, Rutgers University, the University of New Mexico, Southwestern Oklahoma State University, the University of Oklahoma (will petition Board if in unique or special training areas), Oregon State University, Texas Southern University, Texas Tech University (unless in corporate offices, industry or government facilities), the University of Houston, The University of Texas at Austin, Washington State University, and the University of Wyoming (depending on what the practicing state requires).

Will allow appropriate professional degree/experience: the University of Arizona, Samford University, the University of the Pacific–Thomas J. Long, the University of Southern California, Western University of Health Sciences, Nova Southeastern University, the University of Georgia, Purdue University, and the University of Kentucky.

Specific skills, qualifications, expectations, and competences: Samford University, the University of California, Western University of Health Sciences, the University of Connecticut, Mercer University, the University of

Table 4.4 • *School of Pharmacy Requirements (continued)*

Georgia, Idaho State University, the University of Illinois at Chicago, Purdue University, Drake University, University of Iowa, the University of Kentucky and the University of Louisiana at Monroe, Xavier University, the University of Maryland, Massachusetts College of Pharmacy and Health Sciences School of Pharmacy, the University of Mississippi, The University of Nebraska, the University of Buffalo, Union University, the University of North Carolina, Ohio Northern University, Ohio State University, the University of Cincinnati, the University of Toledo, the University of Sciences in Philadelphia, Wilkes University, the Medical University of South Carolina, South Dakota University, Texas Southern University, the University of Houston, The University of Texas at Austin, Hampton University, Virginia Commonwealth University, Washington State University, and the University of Wisconsin.

Strong interest, desire, and willingness to teach: the University of Arizona, Southwestern Oklahoma State University, Ohio Northern University, the Ohio State University, the University of Cincinnati, the University of Toledo, Wilkes University, the Medical University of South Carolina, the University of Washington, and the University of Wisconsin.

Credentials depending on type of practice/rotation: the University of Southern California, the University of Colorado Health Sciences Center, Howard University, the University of Louisiana at Monroe, Union University, the University of Cincinnati, the University of Sciences in Philadelphia, Texas Southern University, The University of Texas at Austin, and Shenandoah University.

Positive student evaluations: the University of Arizona, the University of California, and the University of Sciences in Philadelphia.

Professional organization involvement: the University of California, the University of Southern California, Mercer University (suggested), the University of Georgia, Idaho State University, Purdue University, the University of Louisiana at Monroe, Xavier University, Massachusetts College of Pharmacy and Health Sciences School of Pharmacy, Wayne State University, the University of Mississippi, the University of Nebraska, the Arnold and Marie Schwartz College of Pharmacy and Health Sciences, the University of Buffalo, Union University, the University of North Carolina, Ohio Northern University, the Ohio State University, the University of Cincinnati, the University of Toledo, the University of Pittsburgh, and The University of Texas at Austin.

Continuing education requirements: Mercer University (suggested), the University of Georgia, Idaho State University, Purdue University, Wayne State University, the University of Mississippi, the Arnold and Marie Schwartz College of Pharmacy and Health Sciences, the University of Buffalo, Union University, the University of North Carolina, the University of Pittsburgh, and the University of Houston (three hours).

Preceptor training conferences: the University of Georgia, Purdue University (instructional workshops), St. Louis (community clinical workshop), and Oregon State University (workshops and seminars).

Additional postgraduate training/experience: the University of California, Purdue University, the University of Louisiana at Monroe (clinical preceptors), Wayne State University (certain clerkship), The University of Nebraska (specialty preceptors), the University of Buffalo, and the Medical University of South Carolina.

Meeting with other preceptors and experiential program: Auburn University, Idaho State University, the Arnold and Marie Schwartz College of Pharmacy and Health Sciences, the University of Buffalo, and The University of Texas at Austin.

Specific site expectations: the University of Arizona, the University of California, the University of Illinois at Chicago, St. Louis, the University of Buffalo, and the Medical University of South Carolina.

Site visits: the University of Arkansas for Medical Science, Howard University, Nova Southeastern, the University of Florida, Mercer University, the University of Michigan (some instances), St. Louis, Creighton University (or phone calls), Southwestern Oklahoma State University, the University of Sciences in Philadelphia, and Midwestern University (site specialist).

Follow Board requirements: Palm Beach Atlantic University, the University of Montana, and The University of Texas at Austin.

Selection Preference: the University of North Carolina, and the University of Pittsburgh.

Table 4.4 • *School of Pharmacy Requirements (continued)*

Affiliation Agreement: the University of Arizona, the University of Florida, the University of Louisiana at Monroe (hospital and community preceptors), the University of Maryland Ohio Northern University, and the Medical University of South Carolina.

Survey sheet: Auburn University (self-assessment), the University of Arkansas for Medical Science, Nova Southeastern University, the University of Oklahoma, and the University of Utah (information), the University of Florida and Texas Southern University (biographical sketch), the University of Georgia and the University of Michigan (rotation information), Drake University (practice survey), the University of Maryland, and St. Louis (site information), The University of Texas at Austin (practitioner/faculty profile), Shenandoah University (qualifications), and West Virginia University ("preceptor information form").

Application: Glendale Midwestern University, the University of the Pacific–Thomas J. Long (adjunct faculty), Western University of Health Sciences, the University of Florida (if curriculum vitae is not available), the University of Georgia, Midwestern University, Butler University, the University of Louisiana at Monroe (clinical preceptors), the University of Maryland, the University of Michigan, the University of Mississippi, Creighton University, Nevada College of Pharmacy, the University of New Mexico, the University of Buffalo, Ohio Northern University, the Ohio State University, Temple University, Hampton University, and the University of Wisconsin.

Curriculum Vitae/Resume: Glendale Midwestern University, the University of Arizona, the University of the Pacific–Thomas J. Long (adjunct faculty), Western University of Health Sciences, Nova Southeastern University, the University of Florida, the University of Illinois at Chicago, Butler University, Drake University, the University of Louisiana at Monroe (clinical preceptors), the University of Maryland, the University of Michigan, St. Louis, the University of New Mexico, the University of Buffalo, Ohio Northern University, the Ohio State University, the University of Cincinnati, the University of Oklahoma, the University of Sciences in Philadelphia, the Medical University of South Carolina, the University of Tennessee, Texas Southern University, Texas Tech University, and the University of Utah.

Copy of License: Western University of Health Sciences, Nova Southeastern University, the University of Maryland, and the University of New Mexico.

Letter of Recommendations: the University of Arizona (2), the University of Southern California, the University of Illinois at Chicago, the University of Tennessee (2), The University of Texas at Austin (3), and the University of Utah (3).

Letter of Intent or Interest: the University of Arizona, the University of Arkansas for Medical Science, the University of Mississippi, the University of Tennessee, and the University of Utah.

Additional Information: the University of Minnesota has "Advanced Pharmacy Practice Experience Proposal Packets" that must be completed and returned to a Committee on Experiential Practice for review. St. Louis requires submission of an "outline of expected student activities." The University of New Mexico preceptors that are not in dispensing settings must submit goals and objectives for approval by the Assistant Dean for External Programs. The University of Tennessee requires verification of degree. The University of Rhode Island requires all preceptor sites to sign an "Affiliation Agreement." At West Virginia University, a preceptor must complete University personnel documents to receive an adjunct appointment.

Conducted by the Director of Experiential Education or Chairman Experiential Coordinator: Glendale Midwestern University, the University of Illinois at Chicago,* Ferris State University (or by Pharmacy Practice), St. Louis, and the University of Sciences in Philadelphia (initial approval).

Program director/clerkship coordinator: Temple University and the University of Rhode Island.

Pharmacy Practice Department, Chair, or Dean: the University of Arizona (level of clinical instructor), the University of the Pacific–Thomas J. Long, the University of Connecticut, Ferris State University, the University of Cincinnati (committee for adjunct appointment), the University of Tennessee (vice-chair), The University of Houston (Associate Dean for Practice Programs), University of Utah, University of Wyoming (approves for adjunct faculty appointment), and the University of Arkansas for Medical Science (approves practice site).

Table 4.4 • *School of Pharmacy Requirements (continued)*

Specific Committee: the University of Arizona (level higher than clinical instructor), the University of Michigan, the University of Minnesota, the University of New Mexico, Texas Tech University (core rotations), the University of Buffalo (Pharm.D. Professional Experiential Program).

Tripartite Committee (Dean of Pharmacy, board member, state association member): the University of Mississippi (recommends appointment) and South Dakota State University.

Board of Trustees: the University of Mississippi and University of Wyoming (approves for adjunct faculty appointment).

Faculty: Western University of Health Science, the University of Sciences in Philadelphia (appointment of adjunct faculty position), and West Virginia University.

Continuing Professional Education Department: University of Wyoming (initial).

Reapproval process: Western University of Health Sciences (every two years), University of Mississippi (annually), University of Oklahoma (annually), and Wilkes University.

*Along with the Director of Experiential Education, a coordinator from medicine, community, hospital, and ambulatory practice first determine if the approval process should proceed with a preceptor applicant. If the process continues a contract will be set up and the preceptor applicant must submit the required documents. Adjunct appointment evaluation will then occur to determine preceptor approval.

is not an all-inclusive listing of each institution's requirements/preferences; contact each institution for a complete listing.

Length of Practice

Some pharmacy schools or colleges will require the preceptor to have acquired a certain amount of pharmacy experience before supervising students. This experience may either be general or specific to the area of instruction. **At the University of the Pacific–Thomas J. Long, volunteer preceptors can be appointed immediately, but adjunct faculty preceptors are required to precept for a minimum of two semesters. **It is preferred for Midwestern site specialists to have at least six months of experience. **At Butler University, preceptors must have "at least two years of experience in their areas of expertise, an advanced degree or residency or experience in precepting pharmacy or medical students in experiential education." If the preceptor applicant does not have the experience listed above, he or she is paired with an experienced preceptor for a one-year time period.

At Wilkes University, pharmacists must have at least three years or the equivalent experience of pharmacy practice before precepting students. Preceptors for the University of Mississippi must have at least three years of experience or completion of a residency within the practice area. Preceptors must also have a minimum of six months of practice at the experiential site. At Texas Southern University, The University of Houston, and The University of Texas at Austin, preceptors must have at least one year of experience in the type of practice they will be precepting or six months training in an ASHP-accredited residency program. **There is no specific length of experience, but most University of Utah preceptors have at least one year of experience before they are asked to be preceptors. Washington State University preceptors have at least one year of practice experience defined by Washington Law RCW18.64.011(11).

Documents

This is a section from the chart that encompasses many different requirements. An institution may require only an information sheet about the pharmacist or a more in-depth amount of information may be needed.

Approval

Many pharmacy colleges or schools have an approval process in place for pharmacists wanting to become preceptors. In some cases an approval can be granted after simply completing an application.

Training

Before a pharmacist can precept students, he or she must attend and complete training seminars or programs. This training may be limited to one session, or it can extend to numerous meetings. Auburn University requires completion of a practitioner-educator faculty development program with seminars and self-study. The Florida State Board requires preceptors to "be able to devote time to preceptor training sessions." Since Palm Beach Atlantic University preceptor requirements are based on the pharmacy law, this is considered to be a requirement as well. Midwestern University requires preceptors attend a training program. These programs can either be extensive or basic and are specific to the area of practice.

At Wayne State University, preceptors should either be trained in the instructional methods or have comparable experience to supervise students. All preceptors at the University of Mississippi are required to attend an annual preceptor training program. The University of North Carolina requires completion of the training program within the first two years of entering the experiential program. Texas Southern University has a required preceptor conference for new preceptors. This conference is also attended by continuing preceptors. An additional training conference, the Alverno Model of Task Oriented Social Interaction Assessment, is offered to all preceptors on the topic of effective communication skills with students.

Texas Southern University and The University of Texas at Austin preceptors must complete a three-hour training course that was "developed by a Texas college of pharmacy and offered by an ACPE-approved provider within the previous two years prior to application." At Hampton University, a preceptor training conference must be attended once in a three-year period. In order for Washington State University preceptors to supervise students, they must complete a board-approved training program within the last five years.

Legal Standing

A statement is often made requiring the pharmacist to "be in good standing." Good standing is not defined; however, it can be interpreted as good legal standing. Specific guidelines may also be in place regarding a preceptor's legal standing. Most institutions follow the "good standing" requirements set forth by their board of pharmacy.

Unique Requirements

The regional coordinator must endorse all preceptor applicants at the University of the Pacific–Thomas J. Long. At Nova Southeastern University, the applicant must submit the following information: goals and objectives of each rotation; directions to the site; and a half-page description of the rotation, activities, and site. A person wanting to precept only a required rotation has to send a "letter stating you will follow the College syllabus, including goals and objectives and grading format" instead of submitting goals and objectives for each rotation. The University of Florida requires a clerkship site, a review committee approved syllabus for each rotation, and a submission of "Faculty Workload" document. This document informs the Office of Experiential Program when a preceptor can supervise students.

Preceptor applicants must complete Section III of the "Policy Memorandum" for the University of Georgia. Preceptors and practice sites will be evaluated by assigned students and faculty from the Offices of Experience Programs and Nontraditional Education. Preceptors at Xavier University must also show "tangible evidence of interest in maintaining professional competence" and willingness to meet for lectures, seminars, and workshops. The University of Maryland requires preceptor applicants to complete a "Statement of Moral Character" form.

The University of Michigan Experiential Training Coordinator will conduct a conversation with preceptor applicants to determine what activities the students will be engaged in and if specific objectives can be met.

Students at the University of Missouri are "under the direct supervision of a faculty member." At Southwestern Oklahoma State University, the site where the preceptor is practicing must be licensed with the board and in a contract with the college of pharmacy.

Lake Erie College of Osteopathic Medicine requires that pharmacists, precepting students on advanced core rotations, should be in a clinical position at their site. The University of South Carolina requires initial preceptors to "complete a Memorandum of Understanding," utilize the University's rotation templates to meet criteria for the rotation and develop a syllabus that is to be approved by the Experiential Site Committee, allow the Experiential Director to conduct a site visit and complete Introductory/Advanced Practice Experience forms for available dates and number of students.

Summary

The requirements for preceptors are very different among the institutions of pharmacy. Like the state boards, being a licensed pharmacist is the only criterion that each state has in common. Some institutions have highly structured procedures that are expected of pharmacists wanting to become preceptors. (**Based on 79 of the schools/colleges in the chart as of 3/20/04.) Out of 79 institutions, 73% (58 institutions) have additional specific requirements that must be met in order for an individual to become a preceptor. The requirements vary greatly from one place to the next. About 38% of the institutions listed require that a preceptor have a specific length of experience before supervising students. This length can range from six months to three years. Over 54% of the above institutions listed require completion and submission of some form of documentation from the preceptor applicant. Out of the 79 institutions, 49% have specific approval processes that are conducted. These approval processes may be carried out by one individual or by a special committee. As seen with the state boards of pharmacy, initial preceptor training is a minority requirement among the institutions. Only 25% of the colleges and schools require training before supervision of students can occur. Lastly, legal standing seems to be an area in which most schools just assume the preceptor is in good legal standing. Almost 47% of the institutions listed in Table 4.4 state in their application process that good legal standing is an absolute requirement in order to supervise students.

References

1. Harrison School of Pharmacy, Auburn University: http://pharmacy.auburn.edu/offices/oel/preceptor.htm#Description. Accessed January 2004.
2. Henderson RP. [e-mail]. Birmingham, AL: McWhorter School of Pharmacy, Samford University; February 10, 2004.
3. McAllister D. [e-mail]. Glendale, AZ: College of Pharmacy, Glendale Midwestern University; January 21, 2004.
4. Murphy J. [e-mail]. Tucson, AZ: College of Pharmacy, The University of Arizona; January 20, 2004.
5. College of Pharmacy, University of Arkansas for Medical Science: http://www.uams.edu/cop/departments/experient/ppexp.asp. Accessed January 2004.
6. Winter ME. [e-mail]. CA: School of Pharmacy, University of California at San Francisco; February 11, 2004.
7. Carr-Lopez S. [e-mail]. Stockton, CA: School of Pharmacy & Health Services, University of the Pacific– Thomas J. Long; February 17, 2004.
8. Besinque, K. [e-mail]. Los Angeles, CA: School of Pharmacy, University of Southern California; January 27, 2004.
9. Sylvies R. [e-mail]. Pomona, CA: College of Pharmacy, Western University of Health Sciences; January 22, 2004.
10. Turner C. [e-mail]. Denver, CO: School of Pharmacy, University of Colorado Health Sciences Center; January 21, 2004.
11. Hritcko P. [e-mail]. Storrs Mansfield, CT: School of Pharmacy, University of Connecticut; January 27, 2004.
12. Bunyan WA. [e-mail]. Washington, DC: School of Pharmacy, Howard University, College of Pharmacy, Nursing, and AHS; February 9, 2004.

13. College of Pharmacy and Pharmaceutical Sciences, Florida Agriculture and Mechanical University: http://pharmacy.famu.edu/addpreceptor2.asp. Accessed January 2004.
14. College of Pharmacy, Nova Southeastern University: http://pharmacy.nova.edu/NewWebsite/Documents/Rotation_Form.pdf. Accessed January 2004.
15. School of Pharmacy, Palm Beach Atlantic University: http://cosmas.pbac.edu/pharmacy/Preceptors/Preceptor.asp, Rule 64B16-26.401 and Cheung K. [phone conversation]. West Palm Beach, FL: School of Pharmacy, Palm Beach Atlantic University; February 10, 2004.
16. College of Pharmacy, University of Florida: http://www.cop.ufl.edu/departments/pp/pep/PEPstat.htm. Accessed January 2004.
17. Unterwagner WL. [faxed communication]. Atlanta, GA: Southern School of Pharmacy, Mercer University; January 28, 2004.
18. College of Pharmacy, The University of Georgia: http://www.rx.uga.edu/main/home/experience/Forms/Preceptor/Preceptor%20Application.pdf and http://www.rx.uga.edu/main/home/experience/Preceptors/criteria.pdf. Accessed January 2004.
19. Force WS. [e-mail]. Pocatello, ID: College of Pharmacy, Idaho State University; February, 10, 2004.
20. Cornell S. [phone conversation]. Downers Grove, IL: Chicago College of Pharmacy, Midwestern University; February 5, 2004.
21. Schoen M. [e-mail]. Chicago, IL: College of Pharmacy (M/C 874), University of Illinois at Chicago; February 9, 2004.
22. College of Pharmacy and Health Sciences, Butler University: http://www.butler.edu/utilities/asp/printpage.asp?url=www.butler.edu/cophs/index.asp&pg=226. Accessed January 2004.
23. Shepler B. [e-mail]. West Lafayette, IN: School of Pharmacy and Pharmaceutical Sciences, Purdue University; January 21, 2004.
24. Soltis D. [e-mail]. Des Moines, IA: College of Pharmacy and Health Sciences, Drake University; January 22, 2004.
25. College of Pharmacy, The University of Iowa: http://www.pharmacy.uiowa.edu/CAP/pages/PDFs/IPEIIPreceptorInfoNA.pdf. Accessed January 2004.
26. School of Pharmacy, University of Kansas: http://www.pharm.ku.edu/dean/brochure/degree.html; October 10, 2003 and Kleoppel JW. [e-mail]. Lawrence, KS: School of Pharmacy, University of Kansas; January 14, 2004.
27. College of Pharmacy, University of Kentucky: http://www.uky.edu/Pharmacy/clerkships/faq.html. Accessed January 2004.
28. College of Health Sciences, The University of Louisiana at Monroe: http://rxweb.ulm.edu/pharmacy/Clinical/Advanced%20Practice%20Manual%202003-2004.pdf. Accessed January 2004.
29. College of Pharmacy, Xavier University of Louisiana: http://xuweb.xula.edu/Academic/pharmacy/DCAS-PEP.htm. Accessed January 2004.
30. School of Pharmacy, University of Maryland: http://www.pharmacy.umaryland.edu/elp/forms.htm. Accessed January 2004.
31. Massachusetts College of Pharmacy and Health Sciences School of Pharmacy–Boston: http://www.mcp.edu/ap/sp/pep/proginfo.shtml. Accessed January 2004.

32. Massachusetts College of Pharmacy and Health Sciences School of Pharmacy–Worcester: http://mcphs.edu/ap/sp/spw-dp.shtml. Accessed January 2004.
33. School of Pharmacy, Bouve College of Health Sciences, Northeastern University Massachusetts: http://www.bouve.neu.edu/programs/pharma/index.php. Accessed January 2004.
34. Rider JM. [e-mail]. Big Rapids, MI: College of Pharmacy, Ferris State University; January 20, 2004.
35. Mason NA. [e-mail]. Ann Arbor, MI: College of Pharmacy, The University of Michigan; January 9, 2004.
36. Smith GS. [e-mail]. Detroit, MI: Eugene Applebaum College of Pharmacy & Health Sciences, Wayne State University; January 21, 2004.
37. College of Pharmacy, University of Minnesota: http://www.ahc.umn.edu/ahc_content/colleges/Pharmacy/education/Pharmacy_Professional_Program/Curriculum/Experiential_Education_Program/COP_Advanced_Practice_Experiences/Information_for_Preceptors/Form_Instructions_Fields.pdf and http://www.ahc.umn.edu/ahc_content/colleges/Pharmacy/education/Pharmacy_Professional_Program/index2.cfm?nav=9277&parent=4016&type=F&content_path=colleges/Pharmacy/education/Pharmacy_Professional_Program/Curriculum/Experiential_Education_Program/COP_Advanced_Practice_Experiences/Information_for_Preceptors&content_name=New_Practice_Experience.htm&pic=none&bold=Curriculum. Accessed January 2004.
38. Hoag S. [e-mail]. Duluth, MN: College of Pharmacy, University of Minnesota–Duluth;
39. Haines C. [e-mail]. University, MS: School of Pharmacy, The University of Mississippi; February 9, 2004.
40. Berry T. [e-mail]. St. Louis. MO: St. Louis College of Pharmacy; February 13, 2004.
41. School of Pharmacy, University of Missouri–Kansas City: http://www.umkc.edu/experientialprograms/pharm_d_syllabus.htm. Accessed January 2004.
42. Morin LJ. [e-mail]. Missoula, MT: School of Pharmacy and Allied Health Sciences, The University of Montana; February 9, 2004.
43. Jones RM. [e-mail]. Omaha, NE: School of Pharmacy and Health Professions, Creighton University; February 10, 2004.
44. Augustine SC. [e-mail]. Omaha, NE: College of Pharmacy, University of Nebraska; January 15, 2004.
45. Schwartz AH. [e-mail]. Las Vegas, NV: Nevada College of Pharmacy; January 20, 2004. Available at http://www.nvcp.edu/html/eppe_policies3.htmll. Accessed January 20, 2004.
46. Ernest Mario School of Pharmacy, Rutgers, the State University of New Jersey: http://ruweb.rutgers.edu/catalogs/nb-ug/03-05/pharmacy.pdf. Accessed January 2004.
47. College of Pharmacy, The University of New Mexico: http://hsc.unm.edu/pharmacy/Experiential/experiential.shtml and Denoyer D. [phone conversation]. Albuquerque, NM: College of Pharmacy, The University of New Mexico; February 11, 2004.
48. Schwartz E. [e-mail]. Brooklyn, NY: Arnold and Marie Schwartz College of Pharmacy and Health Sciences; January 21, 2004.
49. College of Pharmacy and Allied Health Professions, St. John's University: http://new.stjohns.edu/academics/undergraduate/pharmacy. Accessed January 2004.
50. Jordan KA. [e-mail]. Buffalo, NY: School of Pharmacy and Pharmaceutical Sciences, Univer-

sity at Buffalo; February 12, 2004.

51. Briceland LL. [e-mail]. Albany, NY: Union University, Albany College of Pharmacy; January 20, 2004.
52. School of Pharmacy, Campbell University: http://sop.campbell.edu/~experiential/pepprogram/preceptor_site.htm. Accessed January 2004.
53. School of Pharmacy, University of North Carolina: http://pharmacy.unc.edu/index.cfm?fuseaction=preceptors.showPreceptorSel. Accessed January 2004.
54. Kearney W. [e-mail]. Fargo, ND: College of Pharmacy, North Dakota State University; January 23, 2004.
55. College of Pharmacy, Ohio Northern University: http://www.onu.edu/pharmacy/experiential/ and document used by all pharmacy institutions in Ohio: Advanced Practice Education Standards for Community Pharmacists Preceptors 09.2002.-UC, ONU, OSU, UT.
56. Cable G. [e-mail]. Columbus, OH: College of Pharmacy, The Ohio State University; January 20, 2004; from Pharmacy 799: Preceptor Guidelines/Standards and Course Core Objectives; and document used by all pharmacy institutions in Ohio: Advanced Practice Education Standards for Community Pharmacists Preceptors 09.2002.-UC, ONU, OSU, UT.
57. Wall AL. [e-mail]. Cincinnati, OH: College of Pharmacy, University of Cincinnati Medical Center; February 10, 2004 and document used by all pharmacy institutions in Ohio: Advanced Practice Education Standards for Community Pharmacists Preceptors 09.2002.-UC, ONU, OSU, UT.
58. College of Pharmacy, The University of Toledo. Document used by all pharmacy institutions in Ohio: Advanced Practice Education Standards for Community Pharmacists Preceptors 09.2002.-UC, ONU, OSU, UT.
59. Cox CF. [e-mail]. Weatherford, OK: School of Pharmacy, Southwestern Oklahoma State University; February 9, 2004.
60. Dennis VC. [e-mail]. Oklahoma City, OK: College of Pharmacy, University of Oklahoma; February 12, 2004.
61. College of Pharmacy, Oregon State University: http://pharmacy.oregonstate.edu/a_level/current_students/experiential/Clerkship-Manual2003-2004.pdf. Accessed January 2004.
62. Mylan School of Pharmacy, Duquesne University Pennsylvania: http://www.pharmacy.duq.edu/srvExpEdu.html. Accessed January 2004.
63. O'Brocta R. [e-mail]. Erie, PA: LECOM School of Pharmacy, Lake Erie College of Osteopathic Medicine Pennsylvania; January 22, 2004.
64. Sheaffer SL. [e-mail]. Philadelphia, PA: Philadelphia College of Pharmacy, University of Sciences in Philadelphia; February 11, 2004.
65. Jacobs MR. [e-mail]. Philadelphia, PA: School of Pharmacy, Temple University of the Commonwealth of Higher Education; February 11, 2004.
66. School of Pharmacy, University of Pittsburgh: http://students.pharmacy.pitt.edu/elp/PEP_Manual.html. Accessed January 2004.
67. Holt-Macey S. [e-mail]. Wilkes-Barre, PA: Nesbitt School of Pharmacy, Wilkes University; February 9, 2004.
68. Spink JT. [e-mail]. Kingston, RI: College of Pharmacy, University of Rhode Island; February 10, 2004.

69. Edwards PF. [e-mail]. Charleston, SC: College of Pharmacy, Medical University of South Carolina; February 12, 2004.
70. Calderon F. [e-mail]. Columbia, SC: College of Pharmacy, University of South Carolina; January 22, 2004. (Protocol was modified from other programs: University of Florida, Campbell, UGA, and Mercer and through the work of the Experiential Committee at USC College of Pharmacy.)
71. College of Pharmacy, South Dakota State University: http://www3.sdstate.edu/ClassLibrary/Page/Information/DataInstances/11715/Files/26566/PartIAPE.pdf. Accessed January 2004.
72. Jones L. [phone conversation]. Memphis, TN: College of Pharmacy, University of Tennessee; February 11, 2004.
73. Offiong C. [phone conversation]. Houston, TX: College of Pharmacy and Health Sciences, Texas Southern University; February 10 and 16, 2004.
74. Collins GC. [e-mail]. Amarillo, TX: School of Pharmacy, Texas Tech University Health Sciences Center; January 20, 2004.
75. Hammond RW. [e-mail]. Houston, TX: College of Pharmacy, University of Houston; January 21, 2004.
76. College of Pharmacy, University of Texas at Austin: http://www.utexas.edu/pharmacy/general/experiential/practitioner/criteria.html. Accessed January 2004.
77. Young B. [e-mail]. Salt Lake City, UT: College of Pharmacy, University of Utah; February 9, 2004.
78. Easton MR. [e-mail]. Hampton, VA: School of Pharmacy, Hampton University; February 10, 2004.
79. Harralson AF. [e-mail]. Winchester, VA: Bernard J. Dunn School of Pharmacy, Shenandoah University; January 21, 2004.
80. Smith WE. [e-mail]. Richmond, VA: School of Pharmacy, Virginia Commonwealth University; January 21, 2004.
81. O'Sullivan T. [e-mail]. Seattle, WA: School of Pharmacy, University of Washington: January 16, 2004 and http://depts.washington.edu/pharmopp/.
82. College of Pharmacy, Washington State University: http://www.pharmacy.wsu.edu/currentstudents/pharmacy%20student%20handbook%202003-04.pdf. Accessed January 2004.
83. See CJ. [e-mail]. Morgantown, WV: School of Pharmacy, West Virginia University; January 16, 2004.
84. Kieser MA. [e-mail] Madison, WI: School of Pharmacy, University of Wisconsin–Madison; January 17, 2004.
85. Thompson LA. [phone conversation]. Laramie, WY: School of Pharmacy, University of Wyoming; February 11, 2004.

Additional Resources

Barnard S, Hughs KT, St. James D. *Writing, Speaking, & Communication Skills for Health Professionals.* New Haven, CT: Yale University Press; 2001.

Gerrard BA, Boniface WJ, Love BH. *Interpersonal Skills for Health Professionals*. Reston, VA: Reston Publishing Company; 1980.

McKeachie WJ. *Teaching Tips: A Guidebook for the Beginning College Teacher.* 8th edition. Lexington, MA: D.C. Health and Company; 1986.

High expectations are the key to everything.

Sam Walton

Chapter 5

Preceptor-Student Relationship

Dana S. Fitzsimmons, Grace M. Kuo, Jennifer R. Myhra

Chapter Outline

In the long run, we only hit what we aim at.

Henry David Thoreau

Establishing an Effective Preceptor-Student Relationship

Grace M. Kuo

Objectives

- To describe the characteristics of an effective preceptor.
- To explain the best teaching style for a preceptor-student relationship.
- To emphasize the need for good communication.

The Preceptor's Professional Characteristics

Effective preceptors have certain characteristics in common. They are enthusiastic, energetic, knowledgeable, self-confident, work well under stress, and are willing to learn. They enjoy their work, freely share information, and seek to further develop their professional skills. They also enjoy teaching and learning from their students. Aware of their duties as professional role models, preceptors inspire students to develop their professional skills and show students how to establish professional relationships.

The Preceptor's Teaching Style

Anthony Grasha[1] has identified five different teaching styles—Expert, Formal Authority, Personal Model, Facilitator, and Delegator—that can be combined in various ways to achieve effective teaching. Similarly, Neal Whitman[2] described two learning styles that could be applied to the practice setting—Pedagogy (teacher-centered) and Andragogy (learner-centered). Because experiential rotations are especially designed for students to develop hands-on clinical skills, experiential teaching is more learner-centered and requires the preceptor to be a model and a facilitator.

A Chinese proverb says "Tell me and I forget. Show me and I remember. Involve me and I understand." A good preceptor demonstrates for the students and involves students in the process of learning. Guiding students to apply their knowledge into practice by having open discussions and competency evaluations facilitates more effective learning for students in the practice setting. Designating specific times weekly for the purpose of reflection can also be helpful. Reflection is a time when the preceptor and students can discuss student feelings of security or insecurity in learning and/or ways of coping with mental stress during the rotation.

The Preceptor's Interaction with Students

To establish a dynamic relationship with students, the preceptor must be willing to invest the time and effort needed to communicate effectively with students. Effective communication requires that the preceptor be sensitive to students' learning needs and be able to evaluate students' strengths and weaknesses without intimidation. Communication is a process, and different communication styles may be needed during the four- or six-week clerkship rotation. Initially, the preceptor may facilitate student learning by giving direct instruction. Gradually, as students become more familiar with the practice setting and more confident in their professional skills, the preceptor could assume the role of a coach, encouraging students to become more actively involved in the clinical practice. Appropriate feedback to students about their performance is essential, especially when preceptors discuss the goals/objectives and the performance expectations of the rotation with students. Preceptors also need to listen to and answer students' questions. Continual open communication will encourage students to keep asking questions and will help them solve problems and make decisions.

A supportive preceptor concentrates his or her energy on bringing out the best potential in trainees. The preceptor communicates clearly about learning objectives and goals; designs interactive learning activities; explains and shares professional information and personal experience; demonstrates skills; provides timely feedback; and encourages continual learning despite failures and imperfections. Though training may involve diligent discipline and growing pains, the preceptor guides student trainees during the difficult stages of the learning process and delights in seeing students become better practitioners. By having respect for their students, preceptors can foster meaningful and lasting professional relationships.

References

1. Grasha A, Richlin L. *Teaching with Style.* Pittsburgh, PA: Alliance Publishers; 1996.
2. Whitman N, Schwenk TL. *Preceptors as Teachers: A Guide to Clinical Teaching.* Salt Lake City: University of Utah School of Medicine; 1984.

Our aspirations are our possibilities.

Samuel Johnson

Roles, Responsibilities, Expectations, and Goals of Preceptors and Students

Jennifer R. Myhra

Objectives

- Determine roles.
- Set mutual goals.
- Define responsibilities.
- Describe expectations.

The preceptor-student relationship can result in truly memorable experiences for both parties. Hopefully, these are affirming memories of professionally rewarding time spent together, although certainly the opposite can be true. And, needless to say, there are all degrees of experiences in between.

What then are the factors that contribute to a positive relationship between students and preceptors? Although they are many and varied, in this section we want to examine those over which the "players"—student, preceptor, facility, and college or school of pharmacy—have some degree of influence. Within any given internship experience and focusing specifically on the preceptor-student interaction, these factors include the following.

Determining Roles

This is an important first step in establishing an effective teaching-learning relationship. It must be clearly understood by both preceptors and students well before the students arrive. The relationship is further advanced when both are comfortable in their roles. Over time and with experience, preceptors move more freely within their role, while students as novices in each new practice site may not be quite so comfortable.

The role of the preceptor is multifaceted. He or she is a teacher, role model, supervisor, evaluator, and mentor to each assigned student. This means that the preceptor must be adaptable to each student that the preceptor comes in contact with (in terms of the student's educational background, personality, and professional aspirations). Additionally, the preceptor was chosen for this role because, among other factors, the preceptor is a competent practitioner. Precepting can be one of the most rewarding professional experiences in which a practitioner engages, but—as a part of a larger array of professional responsibilities—it is also one of the most draining.

Students must clearly understand their role as learners and developing professionals. In most pharmacy curricula, the preceptor-student relationship within the context of the internship constitutes the entire final year of the program. Therefore, both students and preceptors should recognize that teaching and learning are still ongoing during this year.

Students must exhibit and hone professional behaviors during the internship. Hopefully, they have been exposed to professional expectations early on in the pharmacy program and have developed the appropriate behaviors. The internship experiences challenge students to further refine these behaviors. Students should, in essence, "look like" a pharmacist by the end of their experiential program.

Some students will approach the role of learner and blossoming professional enthusiastically, while others will exhibit fear and trepidation. It can be an exhilarating time for students as they try on different areas of practice while moving closer to achieving their educational and professional goals. It can also be a sobering time as students recognize that they have so much more to learn.

Setting Mutual Goals

The success of the preceptor-student relationship is dependent on creating a "win-win" scenario for all of the players. Everyone involved must, therefore, work together to develop mutually agreeable goals.

One mutual goal is the development of competent practitioners through internship experiences. How is this carried out for the mutual benefit of all? For preceptors, it is the personally rewarding experience of assisting the profession's future by educating and training pharmacy students. For students, it is the fulfillment of educational goals and exposure to various careers in pharmacy. The practice facility may view hosting students as a way to preview future employees and recruit students to that particular site. The college or school of pharmacy is able to utilize the talents of enthusiastic, motivated pharmacists and their innovative practices as part of the educational process. The roles and responsibilities of each of the players will differ, but the result is the same—a rewarding personal and professional endeavor and the betterment of the profession.

Defining Responsibilities

It is critical for preceptors and students to be aware of their part in the rotation process. If responsibilities are not defined prior to rotations confusion and chaos may ensue, leading to strained relationships, most notably, between preceptors, facilities, and educational institutions.

Responsibilities should be defined in writing and leave little room for misunderstanding. In many cases, the duties of students and preceptors are spelled out via evaluation forms, course syllabi, and other materials made available by both the university and the facility. Various areas addressed within these documents may include, but are not be limited to, maintenance of official documents such as time sheets and evaluations; observance of due dates for assignments or other paperwork; preceptor preparation for student arrival; student registration for internship courses; student notification of illness; and many others. The responsibilities of the facility and the university and/or college are primarily articulated via educational affiliation agreements, oftentimes developed by entities or departments (regarding legal issues, educational resources, human resources) outside of the groups involved. These agreements can take many months to fully execute. For more information on written agreements, see chapter 7, *Partnerships with Schools.* Periodic meetings between colleges or schools with preceptors can serve as a forum to review each party's responsibilities.

Describing Expectations

Failure to set reasonable and mutually agreeable expectations can result in a disappointing and unfulfilling rotation experience for all involved. Students may feel that their clerkship or externship was not educationally rewarding. Preceptors may feel disappointed if their expectations for student performance are not fully realized. The college or school of pharmacy may feel the strain of unmet expectations from either the preceptor, the students, or both. Over time, this can adversely affect relationships critical to the internship experience.

General expectations, like responsibilities, should be described in some detail through evaluation forms, course syllabi, and other materials. For students, these should be defined for professional behavior as well as performance by both the educational institution and the preceptor. A school-based orientation immediately prior to the internship year, during which course materials are reviewed and students are prepped for the internship, can help accomplish this goal. Preceptors need to know what the college or school of phar-

◆ Preceptor Pearls

- Understand your role in the preceptor-student relationship: as a mentor, facilitator, and role model to students. Remember that the intern's role is still that of a student and not an employee.
- Ensure that the pharmacy and the facility (hospital, community pharmacy, or other entity) have set mutual goals regarding student education within your facility.
- Be aware of the responsibilities of both the student and the preceptor within the rotation experience.
- Familiarize yourself with the expectations that the college or school of pharmacy has described for both students and preceptors. Make sure that students clearly understand your expectations of them within the context of the rotation experience.
- Take advantage of opportunities to meet with colleges or schools of pharmacy to better understand roles, responsibilities, and expectations, and give input when requested.

macy expects from them in the areas of student activities, evaluation, and other aspects of the relationship. This can be achieved within the framework of site visits, periodic group meetings between preceptors and schools, focus groups, etc.

However, differing somewhat from responsibilities, rotation-specific expectations can be individualized between the preceptor and students. Ideally, this would occur immediately prior to the beginning of each rotation in a meeting between the preceptor and students so that both parties are able to make the best use of the time allotted for the experience. The preceptor's expectations of the students can be related to the following areas: daily schedule and when the students can expect to meet with the preceptor throughout the week; specific responsibilities within the institution and how that translates into opportunities for the students; how the students should interact with other pharmacy and institutional personnel; educational and behavioral goals related to the preceptor's practice; and any specific training or orientation required by the facility prior to the beginning of the rotation.

Designing a rotation that meets the students' professional or career expectations can result in a professionally rewarding experience for both preceptor and students. For example, if a student begins a nutrition rotation and articulates an interest in pursuing this specialized area of pharmacy practice, the preceptor and student are well served by exposing the student maximally to appropriate activities and people who can help this student achieve his or her career goal. Another example is the student who begins an institutional rotation with years of experience in making IVs. This student may assist the preceptor with a special project rather than spending hours in IV training, creating a win-win situation for both parties.

As shown above, the preceptor-student relationship is one that can involve a multitude of individuals and groups. Following the steps described above can set all of these parties on the path to a healthy, long-term, and professionally rewarding relationship.

Only those who risk going too far can possibly find out how far one can go.

T.S. Eliot

Motivating and Challenging Students to Enhance Their Performance

Dana S. Fitzsimmons

Objectives

- Examine motivational theory.
- Review the three key issues to motivate students.
- Apply the key issues to students and rotations.

Motivational Theory

What motivates students to act, think, and behave in certain ways? What makes students more likely to work hard, achieve, be creative, and complete assignments? Several early motivation theorists have been studied, and their original theories are still the underpinnings of much of today's modern discussion on this topic. This first group of theorists assumes that all people have needs, expectations, and desires, and that their needs, expectations, and desires must be met if you are to achieve success for your organization (or the rotation in this case). Some of the most popular theories include Maslow's hierarchy of needs theory; Alderfer's ERG theory; McClelland's trichotomy of needs theory; and Herzberg's two-factor theory.[1] Each needs theory differs somewhat in the needs identified and as to how unfulfilled needs influence motivation. Maslow, for example, states that individuals have five needs arranged in a hierarchical format. The most basic needs include physiological needs and safety needs. The next level is belongingness and love, and the higher needs levels include esteem and self-actualization. Herzberg's theory complements Maslow's and describes two types of needs factors. The first type is the *motivator factor,* which satisfies higher-order needs (autonomy, self actualization, self-esteem) and motivates a person to achieve. The second type is the *hygiene factor,* which satisfies lower-order needs (security, social, salary, benefits) and prevents dissatisfaction.

The second group of theories is based on an equity principle. This theory evolved from social comparison theory. Here, people assess their performance and attitudes by comparing both their contribution to work and the benefits they derive from it to the contributions and benefits of a *comparison other.* This *other* may be like or unlike the person (i.e., another classmate with respect to what they are doing in their rotations to achieve success).

Reinforcement is the third type of theory and was prompted by the famous Skinner research. It emphasizes the importance of feedback and rewards in motivating behavior through diverse reinforcement techniques.

And finally, expectancy theory is more comprehensive and integrates many of the elements of needs, equity, and reinforcement theory. Vroom popularized expectancy theory with his model stating that motivation is a function of expectancy, valence, and instrumentality. Expectancy refers to a person's perception of the probability that effort will lead to performance. For example, a person—who believes that if he or she works harder then he or she will produce more—has a high expectation that hard work leads to productivity. *Valence* refers to a person's perception of the value of the projected outcomes (that is, how much the person likes or dislikes receiving those outcomes). *Instrumentality* refers to a person's perception of the probability that certain outcomes (positive or negative) will be attached to performance. For example, the person that sees a link between productivity and greater benefits has high instrumentality.

Application to Student Rotations

Our goal in student rotations is to motivate and challenge students to bring out their best performance. This requires leadership on the part of the preceptor. All students are not at the same point in their development and all students are not at the same motivational level. We want to bring out the best in students by focusing on their behavior and creating consistently high performances. We have to acknowledge that all students will not be outstanding performers, but most students can attain a higher level of achievement. We can use our leadership skills to tap their full potential and get them to perform at higher levels. We create an environment for the student rotation that gives students an advantage to finding the road to success. I will suggest three environmental factors that are under your control that will help you to motivate and challenge your students as well as to enhance their performance. As I discuss these three factors, I will also relate them to the previous theories discussed above.

Develop Positive Expectations with Your Students from the Start

Vroom posited his expectancy theory with the factors of instrumentality, valence, and expectations. You need to take a leadership role from the beginning in helping your students think that they can accomplish their rotation goals. This may not be easy. They interact with many other people, and some of their other contacts may have negative expectations. Positive expectations are not effective in a vacuum. Students have to be communicated to, understood by, and accepted by everyone on the clinical team that will interact with them.

Expecting a lot without having positive expectations of the students is a set-up for failure for both involved. We all know the power of positive expectations with placebos utilized in investigational studies. Think of the placebo that might be used to treat nausea in a study or clinical trial. Now think of the converse situation where a person takes a placebo that he/she has been told will cause nausea. If you have shared negative expectations with your students, they have a head start on failure. And remember the methods of communication that are available to send messages: body language, eye contact, and other nonverbal cues. Make sure that your messages of positive expectation to the students are consistent and match your intentions. Your positive expectations must begin from reality. That is, you must assess the baseline of the students prior to defining expectations for the rotation. This again requires effort and leadership on your part. Once you understand the baseline and accept the reality, your positive expectations can have a significant impact on the performance of your students.

Ensure That Students Take Responsibility for Achieving Their Rotation Goals

You are familiar with the old refrain, that if everyone has responsibility for a goal, then no one has responsibility for the goal. Temptation may be to sit around and wait for someone else to take the lead unless you know that you are accountable, so make sure that assignments and roles are clearly delineated.

Make responsibility a positive endeavor. Do not assign as if it is a punishment but rather as an opportunity and challenge to do something good and to show value and worth. Of course, you need clear goals for students. Do not assume that everyone understands the goals. Setting goals with students creates a proactive environment, which helps students to focus on the endpoint of the work. Without that goal and endpoint, students can get caught up in all of the activity without remembering why they started in the first place. The goal setting session is crucial to students.

Every student is different and you need to use a different style for each student. Your mutually defined goals should match each student's course objectives and abilities. If you set the goals too high, students may become demoralized and fail or give up. If you set the goals too low, students may become disinterested and unmotivated. You can decide at what level you want to set the goals, but be aware that the higher the goals are set, the more you should plan to support the students in reaching those goals. Do not march students out to reach *stretch* or maybe even *bigger stretch* goals without planning to be there for support. You need to think about that during the goal setting stage, and it is probably obvious to you that students will develop faster with your support. There is some validity to the notion that goals should be set somewhere between *too high,* where students will have little likelihood of success, and *too low,* where success is a sure thing. The best goals may be in the area of a high probability of success with challenge still involved.

Ensure that students understand their goals, and ask them to define how you and they will measure success. What is due, when it is due, and what it will look like are all issues that should be in agreement as the rotation begins. Students rarely set out to disappoint their preceptors and mentors—it is often a case of misunderstanding.

Another key piece of responsibility is defining the action steps to success. You do this yourself when you take on big projects. Goals are not reached by pure luck, so also ask your students to do this. Help them define their need to visit the library, gain access to the internet, spend time in a student study group, or participate in daily medical rounds to learn more about their assigned patients. Action steps spell out the big and little steps necessary in reaching rotation-defined goals. A good-action steps document helps ensure success in reaching goals.

Finally, one indirect benefit of all of this activity (assigning responsibility, setting goals, writing action steps), is that it forces students to be interactive, involved, and committed to the rotation. The more involved that students are with planning (with defining responsibilities and identifying goals and action steps), the greater the commitment. Students will know if they are on the right track or if they have fallen off the path and there is need for a correction or adjustment. And the more involved they are, the more responsible they are for the outcomes.

Use Feedback to Motivate Your Students

Be sure to incorporate lots of feedback into student rotations. This will help stimulate, challenge, and motivate your students. Remember that Maslow talks about belongingness, esteem, and self-actualization needs among other needs. Herzberg talks about motivators. Too often students demonstrate appropriate behavior and receive either positive feedback, negative feedback, or no feedback at all. Again, I stress that every student is an individual and different styles of feedback work with different students, and different styles of feedback meet different needs in working with students. All of the feedback information that I will discuss is right from Skinner's theory emphasizing the importance of feedback and rewards in motivating behavior through diverse reinforcement techniques.

Let's discuss positive feedback first. This involves pairing a desired behavior or outcome with positive reinforcement and feedback. Responding with positive feedback encourages students. It is reinforcing and it motivates students for additional achievement.

Negative feedback brings results that are less predictable. With negative feedback, you are acting to stop a behavior or outcome that has already occurred. The result may encourage students to perform better, but it does not always work that way. Students may feel that they are being punished and may quit trying.

Withholding feedback also causes the discontinuation of certain behaviors.

◆ **Preceptor Pearls**

Some best-practice principles on reinforcement include the following:

1. Reinforce promptly; delay diminishes effectiveness.
2. Reinforce incremental improvement; any improvement is positive.
3. Reinforce with attention to detail; generalized feedback is less meaningful.
4. Reinforce changed behaviors and then continue supporting such habits.
5. Reinforce good habits periodically.

Failure to provide positive feedback causes a behavior to cease. Removing positive feedback may contribute to a decline in performance. Withholding feedback may be even more punishing than negative feedback, because it is the least motivating response you can make to any student behavior or performance. And if you ignore a bad performance as if it did not happen, the poor performance is likely to be repeated. Things may even get worse. If you ignore a good performance or even a slightly improved performance, you are going to remove the motivation to improve. Students make additional efforts to improve, and they are not recognized.

Probably the most common type of feedback provided by preceptors is that of withholding feedback, and that is what students dislike the most. Everyone wants attention. Most of us do not recognize how difficult withholding reinforcement can be on students. Sometimes receiving negative reinforcement may even be preferred and may drive students to be recognized in that manner.

A Final Note on Extrinsic Factors and Rewards

Much of this chapter has focused on the intrinsic factors in motivating students. Preceptors are encouraged to develop positive student expectations, invite students to take responsibility for their success, and provide important feedback to students. Do not forget to consider extrinsic factors and utilize extrinsic rewards when appropriate and available. There are simple, inexpensive, and very effective opportunities to help reward and further motivate students. An example might be to invite your students to attend a professional association meeting as your guests. Showing your interest and sharing your time impresses students who look at you as a role model. Also, a simple gift such as a textbook, new health care-related book, or a small gift card provides a strong gesture to students.

Reference

1. Gibson JL, Ivancevich JM, Donnelly JH, et al. *Organizations: Behavior, Structure, Processes.* 6th ed. New York: McGraw Hill/Irwin; 1988:109–31.

The pessimist sees difficulty in every opportunity; an optimist sees the opportunity in every difficulty.

Winston Churchill

Creating an Environment That Promotes a Win-Win Situation for Preceptors and Students

Grace M. Kuo

Objectives

- Create a friendly and helpful environment.
- Understand your role and contributions to your practice site.
- Provide orientation activities.
- Integrate student activities into your daily clinical practice.
- Understand the students' professional and developmental needs during the rotation.

A meaningful, enjoyable, and effective experiential rotation is an arrangement from which both preceptors and students derive the greatest benefit. With careful forethought, preceptors can create a working environment for students that is friendly and fully integrated into the activities of the clinical site.

Creating a Friendly Environment

The professional relationship preceptors have developed with their colleagues helps create a pleasant environment for students. Once preceptors have established credibility in the practice setting and demonstrated value in service, then arranging an experiential rotation for students can be more readily supported by administrators and endorsed by clinical colleagues and office personnel. For example, setting up clinical rotations for pharmacy students in a hospital or an ambulatory care clinic requires that preceptors receive an agreement from administrators or a manager of the pharmacy (or clinic, community site, hospital, or academic department), which grants the time to precept. Often, the pharmacy (or clinic, community site, hospital, or academic department) makes in-kind contributions so preceptors can assume teaching responsibilities in addition to routine duties. Sometimes, the workflow of other colleagues and office personnel is affected. If the rotation requires that students work with a multidisciplinary medical team, preceptors also need to inform the attending physician and make proper arrangements with other team members. Good rapport with medical colleagues and other coworkers is, therefore, the foundation needed to build a successful preceptorship.

After fully integrating preceptor services into a clinical practice, preceptors will clearly understand the needs of the practice site. If the role is not clear to the preceptors, it will be difficult to organize an effective clerkship rotation for students, meet student learning objectives, and provide networking opportunities for students. Every effort should be made to clarify the preceptor role and to identify the needs of the clinic or practice site before a preceptorship is undertaken so that student activities are not perceived as disruptive.

Providing orientation activities for clerkship students is important, not only because it helps the students overcome any fears, but also because it gives students a practical overview of the rotation and the requirements for its completion. As part of these activities, preceptors can arrange a tour of the clinical practice and introduce students to medical colleagues, administrators, and office staff. If possible, a flyer or an e-mail announcement should be distributed to alert everyone in the clinical practice about student rotations. At the start of the rotation, preceptors need to provide clear instructions to students so they can fulfill administrative requirements, such as getting ID badges; computer usernames and passwords; completing Health Insurance Portability and Accountability Act (HIPAA) training modules; and completing human subjects training certification (for those in research rotations). An effective orientation includes the following:

- A checklist that includes orientation items and administrative requirements.
- A policy that covers etiquette and dress codes in the clinical practice.
- A calendar that contains activities and dates of conferences, seminars, and presentations.
- A syllabus that outlines rotation goals, objectives, topics to be covered

during the rotation (e.g., selection of medications for disease-specific management), assignments, and evaluation criteria.

- An initial assessment in which students self-evaluate their skills and state the goals of the rotation. This assessment allows preceptors and students to work together and develop achievable objectives.
- A tour of the office, pharmacy, hospital patient care unit, and/or the clinic. In a clinic, preceptors can have students role-play being patients and go through a mock clinic visit, from waiting in the reception area to getting a medication prescription filled.

Other colleagues or office staff can help preceptors accomplish some orientation tasks. For example, the office staff can help students get an ID badge or obtain computer sign-on privileges. The nursing staff can help students understand clinic flow from the point of check-in to the point of checkout. Helping students become familiar with the clinical practice setting gives staff the opportunity to welcome students into a friendly environment. By understanding the office setting and the clinic flow, students can better assist the office or nursing staff in a busy practice, thus making the friendly environment a win-win situation for both preceptors and students.

Creating a Comfortable Physical Environment

Having a comfortable physical environment will help both preceptors and students attain a better and more efficient workflow. Although many rotation sites have limited office space and workstations, giving students a designated work area promotes teamwork between the preceptor and students, gives students a sense of identity, helps students understand their responsibilities, and makes it easier for preceptors or other staff members to locate students when necessary. Likewise, having a designated desk and a computer obviates logistic inconveniences and streamlines workflow. A work space for students in the vicinity of the pharmacy allows students to be more efficient in providing services to the pharmacy and in completing pharmacy-related or pharmaceutical care-related duties as the rotation progresses.

Creating an Integrated Environment

Once preceptors match the needs of the students with those of the practice site, they can integrate student activities into the clinical practice. The needs of the clinical practice can be assessed by surveying administrators or managers, office staff, and clinical colleagues for ideas and feedback. For example, the administrators may need students to help with outcomes projects related to drug utilization or cost-effectiveness. The nursing staff might benefit from receiving a handout on certain drug information or participating in an in-service conducted by students. The office staff might benefit by having pharmacy students assist with phone calls relating to medication requests or laboratory reports. Other pharmacists or physicians might need help with medical-literature or drug-information computer searches. Pharmacy students might help physician-residents by selecting appropriate medication regimens that are evidence-based and within safety limits. Even though preceptors will need to spend time training students, they can actually help reduce the training workload if preceptors can plan strategically.

Another way of integrating students into clinical practice is to facilitate encounters with actual patients. Treating students with respect and allowing students to participate in a real-time patient encounter, whether in person or on the phone, can help them gain professional self-confidence and, ultimately, reduce a preceptor's workload. Preceptors need to coach and encourage students during initial encounters. Any patient encounter should, of course, be coordinated with colleagues and the clinical staff.

Understanding students' professional-development needs at the time of the rotation can help preceptors design a better rotation program for each student. For example, if a student wants to learn more about case studies, the preceptor can help the student develop skills in this area and even write up formal clinical case reports. Or, if the student wants to learn about research and scientific writing, the preceptor can work with the student to develop research protocols and prepare manuscripts for publication; such a focus requires that the preceptor be knowledgeable about research procedures and have scholarly discipline. If the preceptor at the clinical site offers a residency program for pharmacists, and if the student is interested in pursuing residency training, then the rotation in such an integrated environment can be an opportunity for both to see if they have found a good match.

By following these guidelines, rotations should be a win-win situation for both preceptors and students.

People with goals succeed because they know where they are going.

Earl Nightingale

Chapter 6

Experiential Teaching

Linda Stevens Albrecht, Randy Ball, Diane B. Ginsburg, Christine E. Huls, Grace M. Kuo, Michael Piñón, Ruth Nemire, Kevin Purcell

Chapter Outline

Real success is finding your lifework in the work that you love.

David McCullough

Introductory Rotations

Randy Ball

Objectives

- Explain the purpose of the introductory rotations.
- Define and describe customary introductory rotations.
- Describe the value of summer internships.

Traditionally, pharmacy education has separated didactic, classroom instruction and site-based experiential rotations. The typical pharmacy curriculum has been segmented with the first three years devoted to classroom instruction and labs, followed by a year of experiential rotations. Although some students seek summer internships and others have experience working in a pharmacy, there is no connection between these experiences and the pharmacy curriculum. The result is a lack of progression from these experiences to the fourth-year experiential rotations required by schools.

Required early experiential rotations are now incorporated into the curriculum by some colleges of pharmacy. Other colleges of pharmacy may not include the early rotations within the scheduled curriculum; however, they may require students to obtain a certain number of hours at a practice site prior to the beginning of their fourth professional year. While any experience in a pharmacy can be beneficial to students, early experiential rotations as part of a planned four-year curriculum provides the most benefit to students. These rotations have required objectives that provide a foundation, which is built on during fourth-year rotations.

These introductory rotations may begin as early as the second year of the professional sequence. Although the requirements for these rotations vary from school to school, the intent is the same. These rotations provide students with an earlier introduction to the practice of pharmacy and a foundation of knowledge to build on during fourth-year rotations. These rotations allow students to apply the knowledge they are acquiring through their didactic courses and to see how the material they are learning in class can be applied to benefit patients.

Typical early experiential rotations include basic community, hospital, clinical skills, and ambulatory care. While fourth-year rotations normally require students to complete 240–260 hours over a six-week period, these early experiential rotations are completed while students attend other classes. To balance the students' schedules, these early rotations may only require students to be on site for 16–20 hours per week or 96–120 hours over a six-week rotation period. This requires the preceptor to plan appropriately in order to cover the necessary objectives in a shortened period of time.

The basic community rotation provides an overview and orientation to the daily operations of a community pharmacy. Students may learn dispensing, compounding, purchasing, and regulatory paperwork. Students may be involved in patient education and counseling. This rotation provides the background to allow students to complete an advanced community rotation during their fourth year, focusing more on the management of a community pharmacy.

The basic hospital rotation provides students with an overview of hospital pharmacy, including dispensing, ordering, clinical services, and narcotic control. Students may be involved in journal clubs and may provide educational lectures to pharmacists, technicians, and nurses. This rotation is the precursor to a fourth-year advanced hospital rotation. This will allow students to spend time during the fourth year on topics such as formulary management, sterile products, and continuous improvement activities.

The basic clinical skills rotation provides students the opportunity to learn about clinical pharmacy practice in hospitals, including the review of patients' medical records and lab values. This rotation provides a valuable foundation for all hospital-based clinical rotations that students may complete during their fourth year.

The basic ambulatory rotation, like the basic clinical skills rotation, provides students the opportunity to learn about clinical pharmacy practice in an ambulatory setting. Students learn about the challenges of outpatient medication management and patient compliance. This rotation prepares students for their future ambulatory rotations.

The value of these early experiential rotations becomes evident during the fourth professional year as students begin their clinical rotations. Since students are already familiar with the routine of rotations and the paperwork associated with rotations, students can concentrate on their fourth-year rotations from the first day. Students who have experienced the early rotations are generally more comfortable and better prepared for their fourth year. They have already been exposed to most settings in which they will complete their rotations, and they do not require as extensive of an orientation. The foundation provided by the early experiential rotations allows preceptors to move quickly into the core learning objectives of the rotation. Students who have already been exposed to hospital or clinic charts prior to their fourth year will spend more time learning about pharmacotherapy, clinical interventions, and patient care and less time trying to find information about a patient.

The main potential downside to early experiential rotations falls to the sites and preceptors. Second- and third-year students are not as prepared as fourth-year students, and preceptors and sites must deal with these students differently than with fourth-year students. These students may be on site for half days, requiring a different type of preceptor schedule than traditional rotations. When a site precepts early experiential rotations and traditional rotations, it is somewhat more difficult to balance the schedule.

The expectations for students during early experiential rotations should not be lower than for traditional rotations, but they must be different. The expectations must be in line with how far students have progressed within the professional sequence. These rotations allow for or require more opportunities for mentoring students as the students begin to see how pharmacy is practiced. Although precepting early experiential rotations require changes from the regular rotations, these rotations provide enough payback for the students that they should be steadfastly encouraged. A practice site that provides early experiential rotations and fourth-year rotations can offer a full range of precepting experiences. This is additionally enhanced if residents are present at the site.

Some sites may host summer interns rather than structured early experiential rotations. These interns can be valuable summer help. If the site will adopt an educational focus, these interns can also benefit in a similar way to the structured early experiential rotations. By having preceptors spend time with the interns over the course of the summer, interns will gain a different, broader perspective of pharmacy than they do when they are just being used as summer help. This small investment of time by preceptors can pay dividends for students as they learn more about the practice site and are encouraged to ask questions to enhance their knowledge. The time investment can also benefit the site if students later return for a fourth-year rotation at the site.

Overall, early experiential rotations are a valuable enhancement to the education of pharmacy students. The challenge of balancing schedules and hosting students across the spectrum of pharmacy knowledge levels is well worth the investment of preceptor time.

Destiny is not a matter of chance; it is a matter of choice. It is not a thing to be waited for; it is a thing to be achieved.

Jeremy Kitson

Advanced (Specialty) Experiential Education

Grace M. Kuo, Michael Piñón

Objectives

- Review common principles that guide specialty experiential education.
- Characterize professional and interpersonal skills relating to the practice of pharmacy.
- Describe the impact of teamwork in a successful rotation.
- Explain advanced experiential education goals.
- Provide examples of advanced pharmacy practice areas available for student rotations.
- Describe unique experiential experiences.

Advanced experiential education builds on a solid foundation of general experiential education and extends into more focused areas of expertise. There are many different specialties in which pharmacists can become experts: primary care, intensive or critical care, pediatrics, geriatrics, surgery, infectious diseases, psychiatry, cardiology, gastroenterology, and oncology. Rather than discussing each specialty area, this chapter aims to review common underlying principles that guide specialty experiential education.

There are two main categories of skills that are considered to be fundamental to the practice of clinical pharmacy: professional and interpersonal. The different skills in each category will be described.

Professional Skills

Teach Students to Provide Pharmaceutical Care/Disease Management

During introductory clinical rotations, preceptors teach pharmacy students how to conduct medication interviews, provide patient education, prepare medications with pharmaceutically proper techniques, dispense medications accurately, and ensure medication safety. In advanced experiential rotations, preceptors continue to educate pharmacy trainees in providing patient-focused pharmacist care, which involves the following:

- Evaluating and recommending optimal medication regimens for individual patients (e.g., therapeutic selections).
- Assessing medication effects (e.g., dosage adjustment).
- Assessing side-effects, adverse reactions, or drug interactions.
- Evaluating clinical signs and symptoms (e.g., interview patients for a review of relevant organ systems and perform pertinent physical examinations).
- Interpreting laboratory tests in relation to medication therapy.
- Assessing disease management and adhering to clinical guidelines.
- Evaluating therapeutic goals.
- Monitoring medication therapy (e.g., drug concentration and organ function tests).
- Documenting the clinical encounter (e.g., SOAP note or consultation chart note).
- Billing for pharmaceutical care services.

Specialty experiential education is based on case studies and focused on further development of problem-solving skills. At the start of a rotation, it may be helpful for preceptors to give students an exam that includes patient case studies with medication-specific problems. The students' answers can help preceptors assess their knowledge base and therapeutic understanding and allows them to design educational activities for students accordingly. During the rotation, preceptors can ask students to draft chart notes based on additional patient case studies and to bill for appropriate CPT codes. Toward the end of the rotation, another examination could be given to the students to measure the progress they have made.

Encourage Students to Become Independent Practitioners

The preceptor's aim during a specialty experiential rotation is to teach students how to maintain independent clinical judgment while working as members of the health care team. Students who lack self-confidence and always rely on others to find therapeutic answers will especially need guidance. Assign them tasks with increasing difficulty and give them positive feedback. Students who are overly confident and ignore supervision may need to be reminded to check in with the preceptor and make reports to other team members.

Teach Students to Organize Daily Activities and Manage Time Wisely

As students move from didactic to nondidactic learning and from introductory to advanced experiential clinical rotations, they need to learn to manage their time wisely in order to accomplish an increasing number of tasks. During specialty rotations, they are expected to review more charts, check more prescriptions, evaluate more patients, and document more chart notes—all without compromising the quality of their pharmacy skills. Preceptors can make suggestions to students for maintaining quality job performance based on their own experience and can help them by setting both quantitative and qualitative goals as the rotation progresses. Whatever pharmacy specialty a student may choose, the student needs to understand that efficient organization of daily activities and wise time management are essential to a successful career.

Influence Students to Develop a Healthy Professional Attitude

Preceptors can influence students to develop a healthy professional attitude by being enthusiastic about their work and by demonstrating a strong work ethic. As students are expected to perform a greater number of tasks during their advanced experiential training, they may face greater challenges and stress. As they stretch their capabilities and further develop their professional skills, students may become increasingly frustrated. When this happens, preceptors should not lower the educational standards of the clinical training simply to alleviate student anxiety but rather should explain to students the ways in which they personally cope with stress and frustration.

Having empathy for patients is a professional attribute that can also be further cultivated among pharmacy students through advanced experiential education. As students get more direct interactions with patients and their family members, students may feel more emotionally involved. Preceptors can help students develop professional attitudes that include having empathy and establishing healthy professional relationships with patients rather than being emotionally hampered.

Share with Students the Satisfaction of Professional Growth and Scholarly Development

Specialty education focuses on particular areas of expertise, allowing for concentration in both clinical learning and scholarly development. Preceptors should give students opportunities to help them with a research project, whether it is a health outcomes study, a quality-control study, a translational research project, a pharmacokinetics study, or a control clinical trial. With instruction, students will learn the necessary steps in conducting a research study (e.g., development of research protocols, tools, and instruments; methods of data collection; choice of statistical analyses) or submitting a manuscript for publication in a peer-reviewed journal. They will also benefit from learning about the obstacles that had to be overcome in a research study and will gain satisfaction in knowing that research results can improve patient care. When students observe the enthusiasm that preceptors have for developing scholarly activities and gain some hands-on experience in research projects, they will be inspired to develop their own scholarly agenda.

Teach Students to Teach Others

Teaching students how to teach others is an important component of advanced experiential education. Preceptors can hone the teaching skills of their students in several ways. First, they can allow students to watch them teach. Second, they can explain the teaching techniques they use and describe how they prepare to teach a class. Third, students can be given opportunities to teach through in-service presentations, patient education encounters, and in introductory rotations with other students. Giving students feedback after their presentations will also help them improve their teaching and presentation styles.

Interpersonal Skills

How a pharmacist interacts with other professionals in a multidisciplinary health care setting can affect his or her professional future. Teamwork is essential in such a setting, and preceptors should help students develop the personable, working style that makes teamwork possible. Sometimes this process can be challenging for both preceptors and students, especially if personalities clash. Having the ability to overcome those challenges, however, is important to professional development. During experiential rotations, preceptors can observe and provide feedback to students regarding their interpersonal interactions with other pharmacy staff, other health care professionals, and patients. How well preceptors interact with others in these situations can have far-reaching effects on the future professional performance of their students. For this reason, preceptors should always role model appropriate interpersonal skills.

Advanced Experiential Sites

An important emphasis of the school in the selection of advanced experiential sites should reflect the philosophy of the program. This strategy can help develop student skills in advanced practices to work in a dynamic health care system. Through these experiential rotations, students should progress from student interns to professional pharmacists with the associated responsibilities of accountability.

Advanced Experiential Education Goals

- To develop skills and competency in the advanced pharmacy practice areas of acute patient care, drug information and drug use policy development, ambulatory patient care, and health-system pharmacy management.
- To provide a program designed to enhance student proficiency in providing a higher level of pharmacist care, developed from required, selective, and elective rotations.

- To refine teaching skills of preceptors in both the didactic and experiential training of students.
- To provide a foundation for further training in a pharmacy practice/ specialized residency or fellowship.

Examples of Advanced Experiential Rotations

- Psychiatry
- Pediatrics
- Oncology
- Infectious disease
- Nephrology
- General/trauma surgery
- Drug information/investigational drug services
- Neurosurgery
- Geriatrics
- Cardiology
- Critical care
- OB/maternal/child
- Clinical toxicology
- Clinical research
- Primary/ambulatory care
- Community pharmaceutical care

Unique Experiential Experiences

Pediatric Camps: Diabetic, Hematology/Oncology Hemophilia, Dialysis

Allows students to work in an interdisciplinary environment advising and managing pediatric patients with chronic disease over a one- or two-week time period.

American Association of Colleges of Pharmacy (AACP)

National organization that represents the interests of pharmaceutical education and educators. Alexandria, VA.

American Pharmaceutical Association

Experiences in national association activities and operations, pharmacy practice issues, educational programming, state services, scientific affairs, student affairs, public relations, and project management. Washington, DC.

American Society of Consultant Pharmacists

Provides students with experience and training in federal and state legislative and regulatory processes. Focuses on pharmacy, long-term care, and other current health care issues being considered by federal and state legislative and regulatory bodies. Alexandria, VA.

American Society of Health-System Pharmacists

Experiences in association activities and operations, publications and drug information systems, membership and organizational affairs, governmental affairs, professional and public affairs, student affairs, marketing, and product development. Bethesda, MD.

Drug Topics

Provides experience in medical writing and drug information gathering. This is a six-week program. Montvale, NJ.

IPSF (International Pharmacy Student Federation)

(See IPSF in the site webpages.)

National Naval Medical Center

Located on the National Naval Medical Command campus, the hospital is convenient to numerous educational opportunities such as the National Cancer Institute (NCI) and the Henry M. Jackson Foundation for HIV/AIDS research. As a major teaching site for Navy health care professionals, numerous opportunities exist to interact on all academic and interdisciplinary levels. Bethesda, MD.

St. Jude's Children's Hospital

Hematology/oncology rotation. Memphis, TN.

United States Pharmacopeia

Develops standards for quality of medicines and publishes *USP DI*. Rockville, MD.

U.S. Public Health Service

Bureau of Prisons

Food and Drug Administration

Indian Health Service

National Institutes of Health

There are two ways of spreading light: to be the candle or the mirror that reflects it.

Edith Wharton

Effective Methods, Styles, and Strategies of Teaching and Learning

Christine E. Huls

Objectives

- Incorporate tasks to improve students' oral and written communication skills.
- Create opportunities to evaluate and promote critical thinking, active learning, and clinical judgment.
- Create organizational methods (patient care plans) for practical use by students.
- Utilize instructive feedback methods.
- Prepare students for leadership roles.
- Promote success.

Utilizing tasks related to future employment expectations during student rotations can expand learning opportunities to develop important skills ancillary to job performance. These include oral and written skills, critical thinking, active learning, organizational methods, and leadership. The preceptor's role is to provide a workable schedule of learning opportunities, enthusiasm, a climate conducive to learning, effective feedback, and the necessary tools for success. Tools for success may include folder of readings, online access, library resources, free copying, access to pertinent people, and consistent proctorship throughout the rotation. The preceptor should review student materials, such as journal club article synopsis, and any questions prior to the performance of any task to promote success and a climate conducive for learning and communication. Learning opportunities explored in this chapter include journal club presentation; expanded case presentations with a problem-based care plan and/or mini-review; and university-assigned papers. Effective feedback will also be shared.

Effective Feedback

Effective communication between preceptors and students will set the tone for the rotation and can provide the most important element for success in student learning. Besides elucidating expectations at the beginning of the rotation, one-on-one explanations of the expectations of each experience as it comes up will allay fears and provide a forum for questions. It is most helpful if preceptors provide students with a full explanation of the task along with samples of previous work. Additional meetings with students prior to a presentation will allow both preceptors and students to improve the presentation. In this case, students can be more assured and successful when the task is presented. After presentation of the task, students deserve effective feedback of performance. Preceptors can develop the tool most effective for their site and tasks. One idea is to utilize a presentation tool that divides scoring up into each of four areas, which add up to 100 points: presentation style, presentation content, response to questions, and documentation. Each area's scoring is divided into a range of points. (See Table 6.1 for an example.) Evaluators should be encouraged to write comments that provide specific feedback to students. For example, student comments for presentation style may include "good volume and speed

Table 6.1 • *Presentation Style*

___/15 points		
0–5 points	*Poor*	*Major deficiency in multiple areas of communication (clearness, conciseness, coherence, completeness, preparation, organization, eye contact, facial expression, body language, voice)*
6–10 points	*Fair*	*Major deficiency in one area and minor deficiency in several areas of communication*
11–12 points	*Good*	*Major deficiency in no areas but minor deficiency in several areas of communication*
13–14 points	*Excellent*	*Major deficiency in no areas but minor deficiency in one or two areas of communication*
15 points	*Outstanding*	*No major or minor deficiency in any areas of communication*

of speech, but work on increased eye contact." While still somewhat subjective, this provides a means for a more objective measure of the presentation, which can be collated to a meaningful final evaluation even without evaluator comments. This type of feedback challenges the evaluator to provide beneficial feedback to students over and above the "good job" that may be given without an evaluative tool. In addition, it provides students with effective feedback that they can use for improvement.

Journal Club Presentation

Journal club presentation is a means to add value to the pharmacy department through education, and, at the same time, it provides opportunities for preceptors to discuss such topics as journal club structure and purpose, peer-reviewed journals, literature evaluation, basic statistics, research design, research flaws, counter-detailing, the types of journal articles, reference evaluation, and outcome-based evidence. Readings chosen by preceptors for the student packet should highlight at least some of these topics. Preceptors may choose either a primary research article or a review pertinent to the area of student rotation, be it clinical institutional practice, administration, or ambulatory/community practice. Students should be encouraged to provide a typed synopsis of the article, starting with the citation and utilizing the natural divisions of the journal article. Students should, without fail, include their assessment of the strengths and weaknesses of the article and how this article will affect their practice of pharmacy.

Expanded Patient Case Presentations

Patient case presentations can be expanded to include a problem-based care plan and/or a mini-review. In the institutional setting, this would primarily center on the patient's inpatient problem list; however, this could easily be used in the outpatient setting by utilizing the problems reflected by the patient's outpatient prescription profile. The patient's identifying information should be protected in accordance with current legal requirements and as ethics dictate. When presenting a patient case, students should include patient demographics (age, weight, race, estimated creatinine clearance, body surface area), chief complaint, history of present illness, past medical history, family and social history, allergies, current and pertinent past medication history, pertinent laboratory information and/or physical information (blood pressure, heart rate, temperature, and other information related to problems, such as bowel movement history, change of weight, etc.), and a problem listing. Problems listings should be all-inclusive with the problems listed in order of worst-to-least concerning problem. At this point, the presentation may be concluded with a question and answer time as related to the patient's case. To expand the learning experience, students may be assigned to add to the presentation either a patient care plan or a mini-review of some medication or pathophysiological issue experienced by this patient. Likely, preceptors will need to teach students how to approach a problem-based patient care plan, using the principles of problems, goals, monitoring, and outcomes. Preceptors should emphasize the critical importance of goals and monitoring that are measurable and the dynamic nature of feedback in the care plan.

Editor Role

Whenever the university assigns a paper as a rotation requirement, preceptors can use this as an effective tool in improving students' written communication. Students may benefit from a discussion of drug information procurement and topic selection. Instead of simply grading student papers, students will benefit greatly if preceptors enter into an editorial relationship with students. Staying within the university guidelines for the paper, preceptors can improve paragraph structure and placement; elimination of unnecessary words; use of active rather than passive sentences; scientific writing versus descriptive writing; use of tables and graphs; and proper referencing. With repeated editing over a week, students will develop a paper with a beginning, middle, and end worthy of publishing in the state pharmacy journal. This is a motivator and source of pride for students who plan a residency, fellowship, advanced practice, or academic career. At the very least, this improves the university's student evaluation.

Conclusion

Preceptors can make the volume of work realistic for students by allowing students to concentrate on one main topic during the rotation. For example, in an adult medicine rotation, students may choose hypertension as an area of improvement. The journal club articles, the patients chosen for the student presentations, the patient care plans, the mini-reviews, and the paper revolve around this central topic for improvement. This does not eliminate other important general medicine topics for discussion and learning. It does provide students with one, although rather large, area of reading and studying for their student projects.

Use of these methods cannot fail in moving students along the continuum of improved oral and written communication skills, pharmacy knowledge, active learning, and critical thinking. When students come into the rotation understanding the expectations, appreciating the opportunities of learning and effective feedback, observing the commitment of their preceptor, and realizing their opportunities of success in pharmacy practice, it is a win-win situation for both preceptor and students.

Success in the end erases all the mistakes along the way.

Chinese Proverb

Other Preceptor Responsibilities in the Experiential Education Process

Linda Stevens Albrecht

Objectives

- Determine an appropriate level of supervision of student activities.
- Provide ongoing feedback to students in pharmacy practice experiences.
- Evaluate students in pharmacy practice experiences using summative evaluation methods.
- Avoid common rating errors associated with summative evaluation instruments.

Providing feedback and evaluation of student performance are necessary components of the experiential education process. As practitioners, we are challenged to do this in an environment that places increasing demands on our time. However, our evaluation may be the sole determination of whether or not a student passes or fails a given rotation. This fact instills fear in both preceptors and students. Efficient and effective methods exist to enable preceptors to provide students with useful feedback and evaluation. These methods will enable preceptors to access and guide the student learning process while avoiding errors common to the evaluation process.

Identifying the Appropriate Level of Supervision

Supervision of students in the practice setting is one of the primary responsibilities of preceptors. They should provide enough supervision to ensure patients are not harmed, while at the same time allowing students the opportunity to learn how to perform behaviors on their own. To determine the level of supervision required, consider the following factors:

Background of the Students

Is this the students' first rotation in a clinical setting? Do the students have prior work experience in a similar practice setting? What do the students say about their ability to perform specific behaviors in the practice setting?

The Practice Setting

Is this a practice setting where students will dispense medications directly to patients, or are other health care professionals involved in the medication distribution and administration process? Are the patients in this practice setting more likely to suffer adverse effects due to age or medical condition?

The Nature of the Activity to be Performed

Is the activity simple or complex in nature? Do others have difficulty learning to complete the task? What would be the outcome if the activity were not performed correctly?

As you feel more comfortable with students' abilities, you may lessen your level of supervision. However, always make sure that students have access to you and feel free to ask for your guidance and assistance.

Evaluation of Students

Evaluation of students should be both formative and summative. *Formative evaluation* is prospective in nature. It is aimed at identifying strengths in order to enhance them or to isolate weaknesses in order to correct them. *Summative evaluation* is retrospective in nature and is used to assess competency achievement. Formative evaluation should occur frequently throughout a given rotation. Summative evaluation occurs at the end of a given rotation and usually at least one other time during the rotation.

Formative Feedback (One Minute Praise and Reprimand)

The process of giving formative feedback need not be time-consuming for preceptors. In their book, *The One Minute Manager,* Blanchard and Johnson offer a simple approach to providing formative feedback—*The One Minute Praising* and *The One Minute Reprimand*. Their method can be easily adapted to the preceptor-student environment. Initiate *The One Minute Praising* (Table 6.2) when you catch students performing a desired behavior. Praise student behavior as soon as possible, being very specific about what was done right. Emphasize how the behavior positively impacts patient care or others in the practice setting. A slight pause should follow to let students savor the moment. Then, encourage students to continue this positive behavior.

Unfortunately, it is also a preceptor's responsibility to identify student weaknesses so that they can be corrected. *The One Minute Reprimand* (Table 6.3) offers an effective way for you to carry out this important responsibility. *The One Minute Reprimand* should be initiated as soon as possible after the behavior is identified. However, wait until you are calm and seek a private place to talk with the student. Be very specific about what the student did wrong. Again, it is important to let the student know how his or her behavior impacts patient care or others in the practice site. Although it may be uncomfortable, pause to let the student know how you feel is important. After this pause, assure the student that you are there to help them succeed. You may wish to point out that it is the

Table 6.2 • *The One Minute Praising*

- *Praise the behavior*
- *Do it soon*
- *Be specific about what was done right*
- *Tell the person how you feel*
- *Pause to let them "feel" how good you feel*
- *Encourage more of the same*

Table 6.3 • *The One Minute Reprimand*

- *Reprimand the behavior*
- *Do it soon, but wait until you are calm and in private*
- *Be specific about what was done wrong*
- *Tell the person how you feel*
- *Pause to let them "feel" how you feel*
- *Encourage improvement*

student's behavior that is the focus of the reprimand, not the student personally. Finally, do not dwell on the reprimand. When it is over, it is over.

Summative Evaluation

Summative evaluation is used to assess competency achievement. It is often the primary determination of whether or not students successfully complete a given practice experience. For this reason, it should be done as objectively as possible and with great care and concern. Never take lightly your responsibility to assess student competency. Although it is not easy to fail students, it is what is required if competencies are not achieved. And, your obligation to patients, the profession, and the students demand it.

Timing of Summative Evaluation

Timing of summative evaluation is important and depends on the nature and length of the practice experience as well as the method of evaluation used. In all cases, summative evaluation should be based on specific objectives or competencies established for the practice experience. Discuss these objectives with students at the beginning of the practice experience. Then, tell students when and how they will be evaluated on these competencies. At least some method of summative evaluation should be conducted at the midpoint of the rotation. Students need to know how they are progressing. Make a plan to correct weaknesses that are identified. Do not wait until the end of a practice experience to let students know they are doing poorly. Surprises at the end of the practice experience are never productive for students or preceptors.

Conduct a final summative evaluation at the end of the practice experience. This evaluation should reflect the students' actual ability to achieve the competencies established for the rotation. Resist the temptation to reward or grade students based on improvement. Remember, you are evaluating the students' ability to demonstrate competency in performing specific behaviors, not their ability to show improvement or display effort.

Methods of Summative Evaluation

A number of different methods may be used to conduct summative evaluation.

The method chosen will depend on the nature of the practice experience and the frequency of evaluation. Often, a combination of methods may be used to provide a broader and more accurate assessment of student abilities.

Examination (Written, Oral, Practical)

In the classroom, students are tested primarily through written examination. This method may also be used in the clinical setting. Written exams may be prepared and administered by individual preceptors or, in many cases, are prepared and administered by the college of pharmacy. Use written exams to test knowledge of pharmaceutical calculations, pharmacy laws and regulations, and drug specific information. Written exams may also be used to test student ability to use reference materials to answer specific questions or to provide drug information. Written exams are often part of the final summative evaluation process used to determine a student's grade for the practice experience.

Oral examinations may be a more useful method of summative evaluation in the clinical setting. Use oral examinations to test not only specific drug knowledge, but also students' decision-making and problem-solving abilities. Ask probing questions to ensure students have a thorough understanding of the situation discussed. Alter scenarios or add information to test their ability to reformulate decisions. An oral examination may be used as part of the final summative evaluation process, but it can also be used more informally throughout the practice experience to assess and guide student learning.

Practical examinations allow students to demonstrate their ability in performing very specific, physical behaviors. Use this method to test skills such as sterile and nonsterile compounding, patient counseling, and professional interactions with other health care providers. Establish specific criteria for each behavior or skill and grade according to these criteria. Like oral examinations, this method can be used as part of the final summative evaluation process or throughout the practice experience to assess and guide student learning.

Evaluation Instruments

An evaluation instrument is perhaps the most common method of summative evaluation used to assess student competency in the pharmacy practice setting. Such instruments are usually provided by the college of pharmacy and use a numeric, alphabetic, or Likert scale. Preceptors may be asked to evaluate students' application of knowledge, their technical skills, and their attitudes and personal attributes. By nature, this type of instrument is prone to subjectivity and bias. In addition, you may be asked to evaluate behaviors that occurred several weeks prior to the time of evaluation. You must do all you can to make the evaluation process objective and reflective of student behaviors as they actually occurred. Littlefield and Kleffner have suggested a 5-step approach to completing an evaluation instrument:

1. Observe
2. Record
3. Retrieve
4. Analyze
5. Evaluate

1. *Observe the Students*

   Observe students performing the behaviors to be evaluated. Observe students performing the behaviors at least several times over the evaluation period. Ask others with whom the students interact to observe student behavior. Do they observe the same things you do?

2. *Record Observations*

   Make a record of the behaviors you observe. Do this soon after you observe the behavior. Use index cards or a personal digital assistant (PDA) to make recording of behaviors easy. Abbreviate and use codes, but remember to be specific. Ask others who interact with students to record student behaviors. At this point, do not evaluate behaviors—just record them.

3. *Retrieve Recorded Observations*

   Collect the records of your observations and the observations of others. Sort and organize them as they relate to the competencies to be evaluated. Do this weekly to identify behaviors that have not been observed or need more observation. Use what you learn to guide student learning experiences over the remainder of the rotation.

4. *Analyze Retrieved Observations*

   Look for patterns of performance. Do students consistently perform or fail to perform a specific behavior as required? Do students perform the behavior on their own or do they need assistance and prompting from preceptors or others? Do the recorded behaviors reflect students' typical performance?

5. *Evaluate the Students*

   Use what you learn from step 4 to complete the evaluation instrument. Develop a strategy that works for the type of scale used. For example, if a numeric scale is used, start with the highest ranking and consider whether students have obtained this level of competence. If not, move to the next lower ranking. Continue until you have selected the ranking that best reflects student behavior. If space is provided for comment, describe specific behaviors that support your rating.

No matter what type of rating scale is used, evaluation instruments are subject to error and bias. Familiarity with the types of errors that can occur will help you to avoid them when you evaluate students.

- Error of Harshness and Leniency—A preceptor who assigns a higher rating to a student they like or know well has committed an error of leniency. In some cases, a preceptor may overcompensate for his or her personal feelings toward a student by assigning that student a lower rating.
- Central Tendency—This error occurs when a preceptor avoids giving a student extreme ratings, instead assigning the student ratings in the middle of the rating scale. A preceptor who has little firsthand knowledge of a student's performance in a given competency error may be more likely to commit this error.
- Halo Effect—The halo effect occurs when a preceptor evaluates a competency based on a student's performance in another area. For example, a preceptor may negatively evaluate a student's ability to maintain professional and ethical standards because of the student's poor dress or appearance.

- Logical Error—This error occurs when a preceptor gives similar ratings for competencies that seem related to one another. For example, a preceptor may give a student a high rating in nonsterile compounding because the student received a high rating for sterile compounding. Again, this error may occur more often in cases where a preceptor has little firsthand knowledge of a student's ability in a given competency area.
- Proximity Error—Preceptors who assign similar ratings to competencies that are located next to each other on the evaluation instrument have committed a proximity error.
- Contrast Error—A contrast error occurs when a preceptor rates a student negatively on a competency that the preceptor does extremely well. For example, the preceptor has an exceptional ability to communicate with patients and rates the student negatively on this competency because the student could not perform this function as well as the preceptor.
- Grading on Improvement—This error occurs when a preceptor assigns a rating based on a student's effort or improvement rather than on the student's actual ability to perform the task to the level required.

After you have completed the evaluation instrument, it should be shared with the student. Find a quiet, private place to talk with the student. Review your ratings and comments with the student. Be specific. Provide examples from the observations you recorded that support your ratings. Point out behaviors the student does well in addition to behaviors the student needs to improve. Involve the student in formulating a plan to improve areas of weakness. If necessary, re-evaluate areas of weakness on a weekly basis to ensure improvement as planned.

Secrets of Success

Providing student feedback and evaluation does not have to be a frustrating and overwhelming task. Techniques such as the One Minute Praising and Reprimand allow you to provide students with ongoing feedback in a quick and effective manner. At the beginning of the practice experience, tell students what summative evaluation methods will be used and how their grade will be determined. Remember the process of summative evaluation does not begin at the midpoint or end of the practice experience. Observe and record student behaviors throughout the entire practice experience. Retrieve and analyze these behaviors in order to complete the evaluation instrument. When appropriate use written, oral, and practical examinations to aid in student evaluation. An organized, behavior-focused approach to student evaluation encourages open preceptor-student communication and ensures a less frustrating and fearful experience for both.

Reference

1. Blanchard K, Johnson S. *The One Minute Manager.* New York: The Berkley Publishing Group; 1982.

I am a great believer in luck, and I find the harder I work the more luck I have.

Thomas Jefferson

Potential Precepting Challenges

Diane B. Ginsburg

Objectives

- Discuss the difficulties associated with precepting multiple students.
- Review logistical issues that need to be considered when supervising multiple students.
- Identify practical approaches to facilitate a meaningful learning experience for students.
- Discuss some of the factors that may lead to dysfunctional student behavior.
- Understand why some students may be more challenging than others.
- Identify factors in the practice setting that may contribute to student difficulty.
- Identify strategies for dealing with difficult students and/or situations.

Precepting Multiple Students Concurrently

Experiential rotations differ depending on the type of experience, objectives, and skills that students need to complete and master, as well as where the experience falls during the internship year. Depending on programmatic and state board requirements, it is not uncommon that a preceptor may be assigned more than one student during a rotation period. To ensure that the preceptor provides a meaningful experience for all students under their supervision, some key issues need to be considered.

Difficulties Associated with Precepting Multiple Students

Site Issues

Although a preceptor may want to provide a learning experience to many students, the site itself may not be conducive to having multiple students at one time. Pharmacists are acutely aware of the space limitations that exist in most pharmacies. Many practice sites do not provide areas where students can do research and preparation on assignments if these areas exist at all within the pharmacy walls. Frequently, the students will become additional obstacles to the practitioners trying to provide patient care services. In situations where there is not sufficient room for multiple students, the employees in the area may end up resenting the students' presence as they may feel that the students are constantly in their way. This can have a significant negative impact on the students, as they may be reluctant to engage in discussion and/or ask questions of the other practitioners for fear they may be bothering them. The end result in this type of scenario is that the students may become stunted in their progression and not receive the full benefit out of the rotation.

Workload

Another issue to consider is the amount of work that the students can complete during the rotation. If it is a time a year when the census in the institution and/or the number of prescriptions may be low, the students may become bored and see the experience as a waste of their time. They may compete with each over medication orders and prescriptions coming into the pharmacy for fear they will not complete all of the rotation objectives. For clinical rotations, there may not be enough medical teams for the students to round with, and the medical staff may not want two or more students on a rotation concurrently.

Programmatic and Regulatory Limitations

Depending on the program and state board requirements, there may be limitations on the number of students a preceptor can supervise at one time. Most direct patient care rotations require a 1:1 ratio between preceptor and student so the pharmacist can provide the necessary supervision. This is especially critical during the beginning of the internship year as some students may have less pharmacy experience and require extensive supervision. Some programs have been granted waivers to this requirement and must provide documentation (usually on an annual basis) that the students are receiving adequate supervision and patient care has not been compromised.

Preceptor Time

The role of a preceptor may be one of the most rewarding aspects of your practice. Most pharmacists understand the importance of teaching students and developing future practitioners. Although the desire may be present, a huge consideration is the amount of time preceptors can devote to teaching while performing their professional duties. The level of experience students have prior to entering the rotation has a direct correlation on the amount of time preceptors will need to invest in teaching. Even a student, who has worked in a pharmacy for several years in a technical or supportive capacity, may have significant difficulty transitioning into the professional role of pharmacist intern. If a preceptor has two students with little pharmacy experience, the preceptor's days may be consumed with only teaching and supervising students.

The Success Story Associated with Multiple Student Supervision

If the site, workload, and nature of the practice are conducive, precepting multiple students can positively contribute to student learning. One of the greatest benefits to having multiple students is that the students can be a support mechanism for each other. When there is only one student assigned to a rotation, that student will have no one else to bounce ideas off of and/or to go to for reassurance or support. The premise of "strength in numbers" comes into play here, as the student who is doing a rotation with a colleague will have someone to work with and provide guidance. However, this may set up a somewhat competitive situation. If preceptors are clear from the beginning that each student will be evaluated on his or her own and not in comparison with other students, this potential problem can be alleviated. This can also be beneficial for learning whether the students are from the same or different programs. Students can learn from each other and help each other with assignments and learning the site requirements. This can be beneficial to preceptors as it may lessen the amount of time spent on repeated questions and issues (students may be more inclined to ask their colleague versus their preceptor as to not give the perception that he or she is incompetent). The site can also benefit as the students on rotation may complete many tasks (e.g., drug monographs, P&T Committee reports, drug utilization reviews, etc.). Precep-

◆ **Preceptor Pearls: A Practical Approach to Ensure Success**

- Verify regulatory and programmatic requirements regarding supervision of multiple students. If the environment is truly conducive to teaching multiple students concurrently, work with the program to see if an exemption or waiver may be granted.
- Check your site. Make sure that there is enough room to accommodate multiple students.
- Workload. Make sure that there are enough things for the students to do during the rotation. Request scheduling of students during peak times or when key projects need to be completed (if these can be done with student involvement).
- Confer with and get permission from colleagues. Check with medical staff, pharmacy staff, and any other individuals that the students may need to work with to see if they are comfortable having multiple students concurrently.

tors can schedule certain activities to fall during the rotation period where they know they will have students to complete the tasks. This provides a direct benefit not only to the students in their learning and development, but also to the institution providing the rotation experience.

Precepting multiple students can present both a challenge and opportunity to practice sites and preceptors. To be successful, preceptors must make sure the patient care needs of the practice site are met as well as the experiential requirements for the students. With effective organization, precepting multiple students can provide benefit not only to the practice site, but also to the students in their professional development.

Difficult Students and Situations

When a preceptor decides to take a student on an experiential rotation, the expectations are that the student will work hard and have an excellent learning experience. Unfortunately, sometimes this does not occur. When a preceptor is faced with a difficult student, many times the preceptor may be unsure how to handle the student or situation. In addition, it is not uncommon for a preceptor to blame the student and/or himself for the problems that are occurring. The dangers associated with this type of scenario are that the student may have a negative experience and not pass a rotation and a preceptor may decide to stop teaching students.

Case Scenario

Why Do I Always Get Assigned the Problem Students

Jan is an experienced preceptor who has been precepting students on her internal medicine rotation for years. She was recently assigned a student who had expressed interest in completing a residency in internal medicine after she graduated. Jan was very excited about having this student and had planned specific activities for her student to complete during the rotation. She had even identified some additional projects that she felt would help the student be competitive in securing this type of residency.

During the first week of the rotation, Jan provided a thorough orientation and felt she had clearly expressed her excitement about having the student on her team. Jan went over her expectations and had the student perform a self-assessment of where she thought she was in regards to her clinical knowledge and experience level. Jan was amazed at how high the ratings were but presumed that perhaps this student had done well in previous rotations and truly could perform at this level.

By the end of the first week, Jan was stunned with her student's performance. Her student was not only late reporting to the hospital every morning, but she arrived late for every meeting and left the hospital early three out of the first five days. The attending physician on her team had told her that the student had not followed up on questions that were directed to her during rounds, and that after one week he was not sure it was in the best interest of the patients and learning environment to keep her on the team.

Jan was perplexed and wondered what was happening with this student. She felt she had made things clear during orientation regarding her expectations for the rotation. The student indicated she understood and seemed excited about the rotation. Throughout the weekend she kept feeling it seemed as if every student she had was not performing well and was very unprofessional. None of her colleagues had problems with their students. She wondered to herself whether it was worth it to continue to teach students if they all were going to behave in this manner.

Jan's situation is not something that happens all of the time; however, it is the type of encounter that can have a damaging impact on all involved. Most students are highly motivated and eager to learn.

Why Are Some Students More Difficult Than Others?

There are many reasons why some students may have difficulty during a rotation. When there are problems, the origin of the difficulty usually falls into one or more of the following areas:

- Attitude and motivation
- Attention to their academic program
- Comprehension

Attitudinal Issues

A student that begins a rotation with a poor attitude will present many challenges for the preceptor. For some students, a bad attitude may not have impacted them during the didactic portion of their training. Performing below expectations and being informed that their attitude is poor may come as a surprise to them. Students with this type of attitude frequently disregard instructions from their preceptor (arrives late, does the minimal amount of work, appears lazy) and may become defensive when confronted about their behavior. This student has survived for years with this type of attitude and may feel personally attacked by the preceptor. Lack of motivation is evident in everything this student does (or does not do). The preceptor may have to be repetitive regarding instructions and usually ends up very frustrated.

Even though this type of student may deserve to fail based on attitude, the student may not meet the criteria for failure as outlined by the training program. Students that do the least amount of work possible may still meet the minimal requirements of the rotation and be eligible for a passing grade. This presents a difficult ethical issue for the preceptor and program (i.e., the student meets the minimal requirements for passing but demonstrates a very unprofessional attitude).

Attention to Their Academic Program

Today's students are very different than students from 20 years ago. Many students have already been through the college process, having completed bachelor's and master's degrees prior to entering the pharmacy program. Some students have already spent a significant amount of time in the workforce and are back in college to facilitate a career change. Students may not be as concerned with earning the highest grades in their class as they have other external pressures on them outside of their studies. Students are often married with children or have others to support. Students may be more concerned with making sure they pass their courses and rotation versus trying to excel in all of their efforts. In essence, students do excel in just making it through with the number of things that they have to juggle. It is easy to see how the attention of students today can be pulled in multiple directions and away from their academic program.

Comprehension

A surprising and troubling issue for preceptors is encountering students who perform poorly when they reach the final year of their program. There are two types of students who fit into this category, the *4.0-student* and the *2.0-student*. The 4.0-student may have done well in didactic courses yet cannot apply that knowledge in a real patient care situation. This student may be labeled book smart—knows lots of information but lacks practical application skills. Students that fall into this category may have been able to memorize large amounts of information and regurgitate the information on exams. Integrating this information and applying it to patients who do not present as typical textbook cases can bewilder these students. They are stunned when they are informed that their performance is lacking and that they may not pass their rotation.

The 2.0-student may have worked very hard in the didactic courses but never performed well on exams. Many of these students scored well enough to progress through the program, but their comprehension of information is limited. Now these students may be exposed during their experiential rotations. For some, failure to perform satisfactorily on rotations does not come as a surprise and actually may be a relief. For others, it is not possible to teach four years of pharmacy curricula in a four–six week rotation. Students will end up building on one failure after another and, depending on the circumstances and requirements of their program, may actually be subject to dismissal in the final year of their training.

Practice Setting Issues

For any of the students described above, a busy practice environment can be a prescription for failure. All of these students may be immediately overwhelmed with the pace and expectations of their preceptor and the rotation. From day one, these students may shutdown mentally and emotionally with any type of intervention by the preceptor and/or program. These situations may be compounded if the students are on a rotation with any of their classmates. Even the best preceptor can fall into the trap of comparing students that are from the same program, which only makes the situation that much more difficult for students who are consistently performing below expectations. In addition, students who perform poorly may be intimidated by how well their peers are doing and reluctant to ask for assistance from anyone.

Case Scenario

Why Do I Always Get Assigned the Problem Students (cont.)

After taking the weekend to think through the issues, Jan decides that she will meet with her student first thing Monday morning to discuss some of her concerns regarding problems that have surfaced in the first week of the rotation. Jan tells her student that she is failing to meet the minimal requirements of the rotation on several levels including clinical knowledge and attitude. Her student is shocked! This is the first time she has ever performed unsatisfactorily. Unable to look at the situation in an objective manner, she becomes defensive and informs Jan that she is "just out to get her" and that she has done everything she has been asked. Jan is unsure what to do next and feels that the next five weeks may be the longest she has ever experienced.

Jan thought she approached the student calmly and in a nonthreatening manner. She clearly explained the issues that had arisen: punctuality, failure to follow through with assignments, and lack of clinical knowledge. She was clearly surprised by her student's reaction to the feedback. The student left her office in tears and retreated every time Jan approached her during the day. Jan does not know what she should do additionally to help this student and if it is possible for the successful completion of the rotation.

Strategies for Dealing with Difficult Students and Situations

The first question to ask when presented with this type of situation is "What may be causing the student to perform poorly?" Once the underlying etiology is identified, the preceptor can decide what type of intervention is necessary. In all cases, the program's coordinator at the academic institution should be notified immediately when a student is having problems. The program coordinator is in the best position to advise the preceptor on how to handle the situation. In most cases, the preceptor will be directed to the student's assessment or evaluation form and asked to document the areas where the student is not performing satisfactorily. A comprehensive review and understanding of what the academic program requires and its assessment tool is critical.

Once the problem is identified, the preceptor can institute necessary measures to rectify the problem. In many cases, the student will need to acknowledge the problem before any progress can be made toward resolving the difficulty and moving forward with training.

◆ Preceptor Pearls: Things for a Preceptor to Consider in Difficult Situations

- Did I clearly outline the objectives and expectations for the rotation?
- Does the student have direct patient care responsibilities and can the student continue with the rotation without patient care being compromised?
- Is this the first time the student has been exposed to this type of practice environment?
- Where is the student in the sequence of rotations (i.e., first versus last rotation)?
- Have I been available to provide feedback as the student encounters new and unfamiliar situations?
- Have I been approachable or does the student appear to be afraid to ask questions?
- Do I frequently provide feedback and make time to meet with the student to review progress?
- Have other members of the pharmacy staff been supportive and helpful to the student?

◆ Preceptor Pearls: Guidelines for Meeting with Difficult Students

- Agree on a time to conduct a private meeting. Let students know that the meeting is to discuss a specific issue and is not a routine meeting to assess progress.
- Let students know your perception of the problem at the beginning of the meeting. Try to be objective and clear of what the nature of the problem is and provide examples.
- Let students know the seriousness of the problem. Is the issue something that may cause harm to a patient, the department, and other staff? What are the student implications (e.g., failure of the rotation)?
- Give students an opportunity to digest the news and present their perception of the issue. Is there something that you are unaware of that is preventing them from performing in a satisfactory manner?
- Do not interrupt and/or get defensive when students are talking. This may be the first time they are hearing that there is a problem, and they might need to time to digest the information. It is natural for students to become defensive and emo-

(continued, page 166)

If appropriate, the preceptor should schedule a meeting with the student where issues can be discussed in a nonthreatening environment. This meeting should be held as early as feasible in order to address student difficulties and, when possible, provide time for improvement. It should also occur in private unless the problem warrants having a witness or a member of the academic training program present. Confronting a difficult student or one that is failing is not easy for any preceptor, but delaying the discussion will only feed the problem and not solve it. It is unfair to expect a student to make improvements when the student was not aware of any problems.

The Failing Student

Sometimes students fail no matter how hard a preceptor tries. The mantra to remember when confronted with a student who is having significant difficulty

tional. Allow emotions to surface and give students time to express their emotions and then calm down. Students will not hear one word in a highly emotional state.
- Document your discussion and take notes, if appropriate, when they present their side of the story. This will help you focus on the problem and provide concrete information for resolution of the issue.
- Get student input on how to address the problem. Develop a plan on what needs to be done for successful completion of the rotation.
- Document the plan and have students sign it. This is essential if further action may be required (e.g., assignment of a failing grade, dismissal from the site, etc.). Additionally, having students sign a plan will help them understand the seriousness of the issue.
- Schedule a timeframe for improvement and meetings to monitor progress.
- Thank students for their time and remind them that you are there to assist them.

with a rotation is "preceptors do not assign failing grades, students earn them." Students fail because they are not meeting the requirements of the rotation. Having to give a student a failing grade is very difficult for a preceptor. Even if the student has shown some improvement, there are times when the student should not receive a passing grade and may need to repeat the rotation. The most important factor for the preceptor to consider is this, would I want this student to provide patient care with the type of performance observed? If the answer is "no" this student should not receive a passing grade and be allowed to progress in the program. Preceptors have an essential role in the educational process. The preceptor is the one that has the final say on whether a student is ready to graduate and enter the profession. This is a huge responsibility and one that should not be taken lightly. As much as a preceptor has a responsibility to educate future practitioners, the role in preventing nonqualified individuals from entering practice is as important if not more important.

Case Scenario

Why Do I Always Get Assigned the Problem Students (cont.)

Jan set up several meetings with her student to evaluate her progress and provide feedback. Although the student tried hard to improve, Jan knew that the student had not met the minimal competencies of the rotation. Jan contacted the program coordinator and discussed the student's progress and performance assessment. The program coordinator reassured Jan that sometimes even heroic efforts on the part of the preceptor may result in a student not passing a rotation. Jan asked for guidance on how to inform the student as well as information on what the student needed to do with regards to earning a failing grade.

Jan has just faced every preceptor's worst nightmare, informing a student that he/she will not earn a passing grade in the rotation. It is important to follow the academic program's policies and procedures for handling failing students. Additionally, it is important to document areas where the student has not performed satisfactorily and to provide this information to the program coordinator.

The secret of success is consistency of purpose.

Benjamin Disraeli

Practice Experiences

Diane B. Ginsburg

Objectives

- Identify the different types of practice experiences that are commonly part of experiential training programs.
- Discuss the differences between *required* and *elective* experiences.
- Review internship requirements and types of practice experiences that qualify.

Most colleges and schools of pharmacy have specific requirements for the number and types of rotations students must complete during their final year of training. Additionally, ACPE accreditation guidelines now require some form of early practice training as part of the pharmacy curricula. Where this early practice experience occurs and the number of hours students are required to complete it is state and program specific. Early practice experiences differ from advanced practice experiences both in depth and scope as previously discussed in this chapter.

The difference between practice experiences usually involves a common element. Is there a direct patient care component to the rotation? Rotations requiring students to provide distributive services (dispensing prescriptions, performing prospective drug-use reviews, compounding sterile parenterals, etc.) are usually required rotations for most programs. Additionally, many boards of pharmacy require interns to be under the direct supervision of the preceptor when performing these duties. Most traditional community and institutional pharmacy rotations fall under this category. Depending on the program requirements and student experience prior to entering the final year, students may have the option of placing out of one or both of these rotation experiences by successfully passing a qualifying examination. This provides students with an opportunity to pursue other areas of interest while meeting the requirements of their program.

Today's Pharm.D. curricula requires students to complete several clinical rotations in both the acute care/inpatient and ambulatory care environment. Students will usually complete some form of an internal medicine rotation where they will be exposed to several common disease states (e.g., hypertension, hyperlipidemia, diabetes, asthma, coronary artery disease, etc.). Students may be required to complete this type of rotation in an inpatient and ambulatory area. This is dependent on the program requirements. In addition, other clinical specialties routinely qualify as clinical rotation experiences including, but not limited to, the following: pediatrics, psychiatry, oncology, infectious diseases, critical care, and nutrition support.

Elective rotations may or may not have a direct patient care component. Some programs allow rotations that count as a required rotation to also qualify as an elective rotation. Students may request to have a direct patient care component for all of their rotations depending on their career goals. Other students may have interest in other aspects of pharmacy practice. An elective rotation allows students to pursue their interests while meeting the requirements of the degree program. State boards of pharmacy usually do not count these types of rotations as earned intern hours even though this type of rotation may be required by the academic program. Examples of elective rotations include drug and poison information (although some programs consider this to be a direct patient care rotation if the information provided by students will be used to make a clinical decision for a patient in the institution); pharmaceutical sales and education; association management; legislative and regulatory practice; and academic teaching rotations as well as basic science research.

There are several types of competitive rotation experiences that students may complete as part of their experiential training. Many pharmaceutical companies offer competitive internships to provide students with an interest in the pharmaceutical industry the opportunity to earn degree credits and gain experience. Many of the national and state pharmaceutical organizations offer internships in association management and/or elective rotations. ASHP, APhA, and NACDS currently offer executive residencies. The federal government and armed services have competitive programs for students with rotations at the FDA and the Veteran's Administration as well as within the Public Health Service with the Indian Health Service.

The purpose of life, after all, is to live it, to taste experience to the utmost, to reach out eagerly and without fear for a newer and richer experience.

Eleanor Roosevelt

How To Develop, Implement, Coordinate, and Monitor an Introductory or Advanced Internship Program

Kevin Purcell

Objectives

- To outline an approach for designing a program curriculum and constructing a program manual.
- To provide a framework for delivering an effective orientation process.
- To provide ideas for creating an intern practice model and involving others in experiential training.
- To discuss methods for evaluating the effectiveness and success of a program.

Developing, implementing, coordinating, and monitoring an introductory or advanced internship program at your practice site can be a very exciting, challenging, and fulfilling experience. For those preceptors who have never done this before, the director of experiential education at the pharmacy school and materials developed by the faculty can be great resources. In fact, inviting the director of experiential education to your practice site to see it and discuss the possibilities and school requirements can be a good way to start. Also, networking with more seasoned preceptors is a great way to benefit from the successes and mistakes of others, get some useful tips, and avoid some potential pitfalls. Also, preceptors with a similar internship to the one that you are designing may be willing to share some of the materials that they have developed (e.g., orientation checklist, evaluation forms, program manual).

Designing the Program Curriculum

Designing the program curriculum begins with reviewing the materials provided to you by the pharmacy school with which your practice site is affiliated. For required internship experiences, the pharmacy school should have a course description and syllabus that outlines the course goals and objectives, activities, assignments, textbooks and/or other reading materials, terminal competencies, written and/or oral exams, grading procedures, and relevant course and school policies (e.g., attendance, tardiness, absences, makeup work, dress code, conduct, confidentiality). This information may be packaged into a program manual provided by the school that also contains assignment and presentation guidelines; assessment instruments for the various activities and assignments; weekly hours and activity sheets; site and preceptor evaluation forms; a summative intern evaluation form; important dates; and contact information for the course coordinator and the director of the experiential education program.

For elective internship experiences (especially advanced specialty practice rotations), the school may or may not have a program manual developed. The pharmacy school may only provide the relevant policies related to all internship programs and the required forms that must be completed for any experiential course (e.g., weekly hours and activity sheets, site and preceptor evaluation forms, summative intern evaluation form). In that case, the preceptor will need to define and develop the course goals and objectives, activities, assignments, reading materials, terminal competencies, written and/or oral exams, and grading procedures. Although this can take some time, it is worthwhile if the internship is in demand and will be offered frequently in the future.

Pharmacy schools strive for standardization and consistency in the delivery of the required internship experiences by preceptors at various practice sites. Preceptors adhering to the requirements in the program manual assure that all interns have a similar core experience. However, schools also realize that all preceptors and practice sites are different and have the opportunity to offer unique experiences to interns. Interns can participate in more activities and complete other assignments that the preceptor thinks are important learning experiences. The key is that these unique experiences must be in addition to the activities and assignments required by the school and not a replacement of them. The core curriculum must be maintained but may be supplemented as desired.

Pharmacy schools are usually not as concerned about the standardization and consistency of elective advanced specialty practice internships delivered by preceptors at various sites. This is mainly because these internships are elective and are offered by relatively few preceptors and practice sites. Preceptors are free to build these rotations around their strengths and practice sites and to tailor them to the needs and desires of the interns. However, they still need a course curriculum that is defined prior to the start of the internship so that the expectations are clear (e.g., course goals and objectives, activities, assignments, reading materials, terminal competencies, written and/or oral exams, grading procedures). Additionally, preceptors may be able to improve their elective advanced specialty practice internship by working together with preceptors of similar elective rotations and sharing and combining the ideas and materials developed by each other.

Constructing the Program Manual

Many preceptors use the program manual provided to them by the pharmacy school, which is perfectly appropriate. Some preceptors take the school's program manual and incorporate it into a more comprehensive program manual that they have customized for their rotation and practice site (a real "survival manual"). All the materials can be placed into a three-ring binder that has tabs dividing the sections. Table 6.4 lists example components that could be included in a program manual. By developing a program manual, preceptors can use their creativity and express themselves in a way that might facilitate building a good preceptor-intern relationship and decrease the initial anxiety of the intern. This also is an opportunity for preceptors to reveal their artistic side and their sense of humor as well as demonstrate their commitment, enthusiasm, and forethought.

Conducting an Effective Orientation Process

The orientation process is critically important since it becomes part of the intern's first impression of the preceptor and the practice site, and it can set the

Table 6.4 • *Example Components for a Program Manual*

- *Welcome letter*
- *Diagram and directory of the health care organization*
- *Map and guide for the area*
- *Orientation checklist*
- *Forms that must be completed (e.g., self-assessment, hours sheet, practice site evaluation, preceptor evaluation, intern evaluation)*
- *Copy of state regulations related to intern duties*
- *Brief biographical statements about the preceptors*
- *List of the names of all pharmacy employees and their positions*
- *Brief description of the pharmacy department and the health care organization*
- *Copies of the Pledge of Professionalism, Oath of a Pharmacist, and Code of Ethics for Pharmacists*
- *Goals and objectives of the internship*
- *Competencies that must be demonstrated*
- *Required activities, assignments, and exams*
- *Copies of articles or presentations to read and discuss*
- *Sample assignment write-ups (e.g., research papers, formulary monographs, case studies, clinical intervention reports), problem sets, and exam questions*
- *Example formats for organizing oral presentations (e.g., patient cases, journal articles, in-services) and patient care notes (e.g., medication and allergy histories, progress notes, consultations)*
- *Detailed schedule showing all the important activities and deadlines for assignments*
- *Cartoons and jokes*
- *Inspirational stories*
- *Art and history relevant to pharmacy*
- *Anything else that you want to share with the intern to show your personality, to make learning fun, and to enhance the intern's transition and experience at your practice site*

tone for the rest of the internship. The orientation process may begin before the intern arrives at the practice site on the first day. The preceptor and intern can have a brief conversation prior to the rotation. Essential information to be communicated includes directions to the health care organization, parking, arrival time, meeting place, and contact information for the preceptor in case of mishap (e.g., intern is lost, has an accident, or gets sick). Also, this is a chance for the preceptor to ask a few questions and allay any fears or misconceptions the intern has. The orientation process should resume as early as possible on the first day of the internship. A checklist can be used to guide the orientation process and make sure nothing is left out. Table 6.5 lists example items that could be included in an orientation checklist. If the orientation process cannot occur immediately after the intern's arrival because the preceptor has become unexpectedly busy, the intern can shadow the preceptor until things slow down and time can be made. Having interns come back later that day or the next day sends a bad message about the preceptor's level of commitment. Conducting an

Table 6.5 • *Example Items for an Orientation Checklist*

- *Verify that intern's license/registration is current*
- *Discuss background, pharmacy experience, and career goals and plans of the intern and preceptor*
- *Discuss expectations of the intern and preceptor (e.g., conduct, ethics, confidentiality)*
- *Discuss any unique needs of the intern (e.g., health, religious)*
- *Tour the pharmacy and point out important areas (e.g., work space, break room, phone, bathroom, references)*
- *Meet the preceptors and other pharmacy staff*
- *Tour the rest of practice site and meet other key people*
- *Obtain name badge and clearance codes (e.g., pharmacy, library, and computer access) and complete any other processing requirements of the health care organization (e.g. review immunization records)*
- *Review pertinent policy and procedure of the pharmacy department and the health care organization (e.g., dress code, phone use, universal precautions)*
- *Review the internship program manual*
- *Clarify the pharmacy duties and responsibilities that the intern will be held accountable for doing*
- *Discuss the required activities and assignments and their completion dates*
- *Clarify the schedules of the intern and preceptors*
- *Discuss the feedback and evaluation process*
- *Provide contact information for the preceptors (e.g., work phone, pager, e-mail, home phone)*

effective orientation process can begin the development of a good preceptor-intern relationship and start off the internship on a positive note.

Creating an Intern Practice Model and Assigning Duties and Responsibilities

Interns know when they are doing "busy work" that is not important to the operational mission of the pharmacy and that keeps them out of the way of the preceptors. Being sent off to work on these exercises of futility (e.g., constructing forms or pamphlets that will never be used by the pharmacy) can be very frustrating to them. Interns like to be engaged in meaningful work that allows them to contribute to the pharmacy, learn new things, and grow and develop as pharmacists.

One way to assure that interns are engaged in meaningful work is to create an intern practice model with designated duties and responsibilities that they will be held accountable for completing. Depending on the type of internship and practice site, these duties and responsibilities may be related to drug distribution services, clinical pharmacy services, a blend of both, or other types of services. Assigned tasks may be constant over the course of an internship or they may change as interns are rotated to different areas or are given progressive levels of duties and responsibilities. In every case, it is important to explain to them why each task is important and what knowledge, skills, and terminal competencies you expect them to gain from doing it.

Potential duties and responsibilities that could be included in an intern practice model are listed in Table 6.6. When constructing a list of duties and responsibilities for an intern practice model, think in terms of the types of things you would want an entry-level pharmacist who was just employed by your health care organization to be able to do. Also, think about activities that would be good learning experiences for interns and at the same time would expand or improve the services offered by your pharmacy.

Involving Pharmacy Staff and Other Health Care Professionals and Patients in Experiential Training

Many people can be involved in various aspects in the training of interns. Inclusion of people other than the primary preceptor is usually dependent on

Table 6.6• *Potential Duties and Responsibilities for an Intern Practice Model*

- *Ordering drugs and stocking them on the shelves*
- *Taking new prescriptions and transferring prescriptions over the phone*
- *Preparing, labeling, and dispensing prescriptions*
- *Obtaining medication and allergy histories from patients and documenting them in the medical record*
- *Answering drug information questions from patients or other health care professionals*
- *Triaging patients and assisting them with the selection of over-the-counter products*
- *Performing patient counseling related to medications and devices and documenting it in the medical record*
- *Conducting drug regimen reviews for all patients on the assigned patient care unit*
- *Seeing patients every day on the assigned patient care unit and assessing their subjective and objective responses to medication therapy, including performing therapeutic drug monitoring as needed*
- *Making recommendations to physicians related to drug therapy and working with them on developing the pharmacotherapy portion of the patient care plan*
- *Writing progress notes and/or consultation notes as appropriate*
- *Serving as a liaison for the pharmacy department on the assigned patient care unit*
- *Providing in-services to the pharmacy and nursing staff on requested or targeted topics*

the type of rotation, the kind of practice site, and the desire of others to teach. Pharmacy technicians, staff pharmacists, clinical pharmacists, pharmacy managers, nurses, nurse practitioners, physician assistants, respiratory therapists, dietitians, and physicians are among those who frequently participate. Interns can spend some time with different health care professionals in order to get exposed to certain areas or to focus on learning specific skills. For example, interns can learn first hand about issues related to medication administration techniques and devices (e.g., infusion pumps) by working with nurses. Interns can enhance their patient assessment and physical examination skills through working with physicians, nurse practitioners, and physician assistants. Interns can sharpen their patient counseling skills related to use of a nebulizer, inhaler, and peak flow meter by working with a respiratory therapist or related to nutrition by working with a dietitian. These other health care professionals can provide feedback to the primary preceptor about the intern's performance and, thus, contribute to the evaluation process.

Patients can also be involved in the training of interns, particularly in the evaluation process. Although patients may not be able to assess an intern's pharmacy knowledge or technical skills, they can evaluate an intern's professionalism, communication and listening ability, and interpersonal skills. Preceptors can have patients fill out a very short and simple intern assessment form after their interaction with an intern. The form should contain no more than a handful of items to evaluate and fit on one piece of paper or an oversized index card. Patients may be very happy to play a small role like this in the education and training of future pharmacists. Patients also can be involved in more complex competency assessment methods, such as practical exams (objective structured clinical exams), and they can be taught to give verbal feedback directly to the interns.

Evaluating the Effectiveness and Success of the Program

Pharmacy schools should be able to provide preceptors with evaluation summaries of their internship program and their practice site on a periodic basis (e.g., annually). How often this occurs may be dependent on how frequently students complete an internship with the preceptor at a given practice site. Schools are always concerned about maintaining student anonymity, which can be important in getting valid evaluations. Also, most schools have hundreds of preceptors and practice sites but few personnel devoted to experiential education that can compile and send out evaluation summaries. Unfortunately, preceptors cannot improve themselves, their internship, or their practice site without valuable and timely feedback.

If preceptors are not receiving evaluation summaries from the pharmacy school on a regular basis, they can develop their own preceptor, internship, and practice site evaluation forms. These can be distributed, completed, and turned in during the last day of the rotation after the interns have received their final grade. Also, preceptors can conduct exit interviews with the interns at the end of their last day, discuss the evaluations with them, and seek additional verbal feedback. Interns usually are very willing to do this if they have been told that it is solely for continuous quality improvement purposes so that the preceptor, internship, and practice site can be improved.

Besides reviewing evaluation summaries and setting goals in terms of the scores, there may be some other metrics that can be tracked to evaluate the effectiveness and success of the internship program. These metrics will be dependent on the goals the preceptor and his/her supervisor have for the internship program. Often the primary goal of the internship program is to improve the recruitment of pharmacy residents and/or pharmacists. The number of positions filed by graduates from the affiliated pharmacy school can be tracked over time. A secondary goal may be to improve the job satisfaction and retention of pharmacists by making their work more intrinsically rewarding, which can be evaluated through repeated surveys. Other indirect measures of success that could be tracked include the number of requests made per year by students to complete a required or elective internship at the practice site; the number of pharmacy schools forming partnerships with the practice site; and the total number of interns trained per year. Of course, receiving invitations to speak at school-sponsored preceptor conferences and being presented with preceptor awards would be signs of success for those desiring to become master preceptors.

The achievement of one goal should be the starting point of another.

Alexander Graham Bell

Essential Components of a Continuous Quality Improvement Process for Your Experiential Training Program

Ruth Nemire

Objective

- To define continuous quality improvement as it relates to experiential training programs.

The concept of accreditation is not new to most pharmacy practitioners because institutions are judged on performance and continue to exist because they meet standards set up by some national accrediting organization. Accreditation councils oversee organizations and institutions to make sure that they are operating in ways that meet at least a minimum standard. The Accreditation Council for Pharmacy Education (ACPE) is the national accrediting body for colleges and schools of pharmacy. It is in place to measure the minimum standards by which pharmacy schools function.[1] ACPE acts as a judge of the quality of a pharmacy school program, and they, in turn, expect that each college should have its own standards and ways of assessing programs and faculty to ensure that minimum educational and program standards are met.

There are many definitions of continuous quality improvement (CQI). Here are three definitions from the American Society for Quality, The Delaware Healthcare Association, and the Mental Health Association of Ohio. One of them should work for just about any training program.

1. "Philosophy and attitude for analyzing capabilities and processes and improving them repeatedly to achieve the objective of customer satisfaction."[2]

2. "Process to continuously make everything better each day. The initiative is customer focused and requires that processes be analyzed, measured, improved and evaluated on an ongoing basis."[3]
3. "Ongoing betterment of products, services or processes through incremental and breakthrough enhancements."[4]

The key point that every definition contains is that the process is continuous in developing ways to improve a program. The organization involved in training students may have a continuous quality improvement definition in place, which is appropriate to use. Many colleges of pharmacy have one or more committees to evaluate and assess the curriculum and the programs offered. The committee or task force that most likely will impact the preceptor is one that functions from the Department of Pharmacy Practice or the Office of Experiential Education. The administration and faculty in the practice department are most concerned with what is happening at the training sites concerning both student training and availability of tools for students to practice skills. A committee may be called the Continuous Quality Improvement (CQI) committee, or the Experiential Education Programs Assessment (EPAC) committee, or a variety of other names. The responsibilities of this committee are to evaluate and assess practice sites, preceptors, and the program at a site. Members will be looking at technology, the number of people involved in the program, the training of the individuals involved in the program, and opportunities available for student training (Table 6.7).

These committees take into account assessments from students, assessments from peers, personal interactions with the preceptors at the site, and involvement of preceptors in college or school training programs. Most schools and colleges have students complete an evaluation form that includes information about the site, and/or the preceptor, and/or the program. The information contained in these forms is often shared directly with preceptors in a way that provides anonymous feedback. One way a school or faculty member may evaluate the quality of a site is by the interaction of the preceptors with the school as this may be a reflection of how students are treated. Sites and preceptors who continuously back out of commitments to students are not perceived as quality

Table 6.7 • Continuous Quality Improvement—What a School is Looking For

Site	Preceptor	Site Program
Meets accrediting body standards if applicable *Accessible to students and faculty* *Maintains technology in pharmacy* *Maintains and provides technology to students in order to meet the demands of the course (computer, etc.).* *Administrative support for student training programs*	*Licensed, meets State Board standards for providing training to students* *Has a plan for training students* *Has technology to meet the needs of the College or School of Pharmacy* *Has appropriate training and/or experience to provide the opportunities to meet goals and objectives of course maintained by college or school* *Has contingency plans in place to cover primary preceptor absences* *Is internally motivated to provide educational opportunities* *Responsive to representative from college or school*	*Provides students with multiple opportunities to meet select course goals and objectives* *Multiple disciplines involved in training program* *Incorporates the use of technology for student learning* *Incorporates group discussions and peer interaction among all students during concurrent training times* *Provides reflection opportunities for students and preceptors*

sites for placement. All of the criteria listed in the Table 6.7 should be considered when developing your training program for students.

Whether you as a preceptor or a team from the pharmacy department decide to develop a quality assurance or continuous improvement program, four elements of evaluation and assessment should be included: peer, student, college, and other health care professionals (Table 6.8). Peer assessment comes in the form of those around you who may also work with students or who view your interactions with students. Developing a form similar to one used by human resources departments may provide an indication to you of how others view your performance with students. You should also complete a preceptor self-evaluation each year, or after several students complete their evaluations, to see how you think you are doing. This will provide you with quantitative feedback to compare when you get assessments from other individuals.

College assessment is not always limited to—but may only be provided in—

the form of student evaluations. College assessment committees may also provide an annual or periodic review by sending a faculty member to the site to look around and inquire about the program. This assessment by the college or school may just be a phone call to get your input. There are over 90 colleges and schools of pharmacy in the United States and each will operate a little differently. When seeking to participate with the college training program, a preceptor should ask how they will be evaluated and what quality assurance measures the college has set forth. Other health care providers who may or may not be involved in your specific training program will be able to provide feedback because they have had interactions with students and may have watched you interact. The feedback they provide may help improve the training program logistically or programmatically. Also, getting feedback from other health professionals may help to draw them into the program either as a preceptor or as an individual who helps you train the students.

Finally, while all courses do not involve direct patient care, those that do could include patients in their quality assurance or improvement measures. Patients can provide a lot of helpful feedback regarding student performance, including how they were treated. Patients may accept certain services from students that you, as a preceptor, may not have considered. Many patients are eager to participate in a program where they feel they are getting one-on-one attention, even if it is a training program. Some patients may be hesitant in participating, but even those who are not interested can provide feedback on why they do not wish to participate.

Consider developing a continuous, quality improvement program as an extension of your practice, in either an operative or patient care practice. Continuous quality improvement should fit into your daily routine and should not require great amounts of extra work. If it does, then you have not set up the program correctly and should reflect and reevaluate the needs of your quality improvement process.

Involving All Pharmacy Staff Members, Other Health Care Professionals, and Patients in Experiential Training

It is important to involve all members of the pharmacy department in training students, not just one individual. Familiarize staff members with students goals

Table 6.8 • *Where to Get Assessment and Evaluations of the Site, Preceptor, and Program*

Peer Assessment: *Provides you with information that you can not see yourself about the training program and about your actions. Develop an evaluation form such as those used for performance evaluation.*
Student Feedback: *May provide you with both constructive feedback as well as comments that may cause you to think twice about taking students, but in the end may help improve the performance of the site and those interacting with students.*
College Feedback: *This feedback may come from student evaluations or from interactions and may be valuable in helping change the logistics of the course at the site, or in students' perception of the course and site.*
Feedback from Other HP: *Other health care professionals can provide feedback about student performance as well as logistical assessment of the program provided by your site.*
Patients (if applicable): *The patient always has something to discuss about a student or about how a student was presented to them and timetables. Include patient evaluations of students, or logistics, or what patients would like to see in a program developed when possible.*

and objectives as well as the roles that everyone will play in training. Staff involvement can help reduce the workload and stress that is often caused by the introduction of students into a pharmacy. This is one of the most important aspects in starting or continuing an experiential training program.

Anyone who is going to be involved in student training (Table 6.9) should be recognized as a preceptor in some capacity, whether it is the pharmacy administration and/or the pharmacist. It increases the commitment to the program, and students become more accepting when that recognition exists. Who can be a preceptor is an age-old question for many. Students are going to be in contact with many people who will provide them with various amounts of skills training and information. At the very least, pharmacists and technicians in the pharmacy should be recognized and involved in the training program.

Technicians often spend a lot of time with students, teaching them the technical skills they need to be pharmacists. The recognition of that fact is very important, especially when students do not view the technician's role as

Table 6.9 • *Who Can Participate and What They Can Do with the Students*

Preceptor	*Coordinate the logistics of course, rounding, journal clubs, projects, feedback and assessment, general practice skills-patient or nondirect patient care oriented, presentations, acclimation to the profession, site and other health care professionals, integration of knowledge and skills in practice*
Other Pharmacists	*General practice skills-patient or nondirect patient care oriented, journal clubs, presentations, acclimation to the profession, site and other health care professionals, integration of knowledge and skills in practice*
Technicians	*General practice techniques and skills, acclimation to the site, introductions, rules and regulations*
Management/ Administrative Staff	*General business and operational/management skills, business rules and regulations, acclimation to the site*
Physicians	*Diagnostic procedures, physical assessment, communication and professional interaction, integration of knowledge and skills in practice*
Nursing	*Logistics, what's in a chart, where to find the charts, specific patient care, physical assessment and medication administration, and management logistics*
X-ray Physicians	*Expose the students to the x-rays so they understand what they are looking at, or what the diagnosis means when they read an x-ray report*
Hematology Laboratory Administration and Staff	*Expose the students to the laboratory procedures, the lab panels at the site, the normals, abnormals, and what drugs interfere with testing*
Patients	*Inpatient or outpatient settings, develop and improve communication skills, understanding of disease state outcomes, medications, drug interactions, and adherence*

valuable to them in their learning process. This is a scenario within the pharmacy that can be avoided if technicians are taught about student roles, goals and objectives, and activities required for various courses. Technicians also need to know what their own roles and duties are in student training. The technical staff can train students in the day-to-day operational skills required in the pharmacy—from filling carts, to delivering medications, to the IV room function, and the daily ordering processes. For students who have never been in a hospital before, assigning them duties with the head technician for a period of time is not unreasonable. Once students have been exposed to the technical duties required in a hospital, they can move on to the duties of a pharmacist.

All pharmacists who are going to be involved with students need to be aware of their own roles as well as the goals and objectives of the students (Table 6.10). This is the case for all of the health care professionals involved in the program. It is a good idea to set up an organizational meeting and an annual meeting for those taking responsibility for students. Announce which schools

Table 6.10 • *When You are the Primary Preceptor and Are Involving Others in the Training Program*

Do	Do NOT
• *Explain their role and their authority with students to the person you are enlisting to help* • *Explain that the students are taking a course* • *Discuss the goal and objectives of the course* • *Explain the student responsibilities to the site* • *Include them in the orientation program for students* • *Schedule their time with students* • *Provide them with a copy of the evaluation tool used by the college* • *Get feedback from them on student performance* • *Provide them with feedback from students about their performance*	• *Dump students in their office or work area* • *Ask someone to help without providing the list of Do's in the left hand column* • *Provide just the manual* • *Say "You know what to do"* • *Exclude them from the orientation process* • *Forget to tell them when they will be helping with students* • *Forget to show them how the students are evaluated* • *Forget to get feedback or ignore their feedback on student performance* • *Ignore their performance with students*

◆ **PRECEPTOR PEARLS**

What to Do for Students Before and during the Experiential Course

Do

- Provide an in-depth orientation
- Introduce the students to administrative personnel, pharmacists, support staff, nursing staff, physicians, other leaders
- Cover the area of responsibilities for the students
- Cover the areas of responsibilities for the staff and pharmacists
- Provide the students with a course schedule including activities and due dates
- Help the students reflect often on activities and the learning that has occurred
- Provide a site map if available
- Provide the emergency number on site for security

(continued, page 187

will be sending students. In this meeting, the kind of students who will be assigned to the site should be addressed. Many schools of pharmacy have implemented introductory practice experience courses; consequently, not all students who attend a site for training are in their last year. Plan a course with the pharmacists, technicians, and any other health care providers who will be involved in the training program. In the end, a schedule should be developed that includes the days and activities as well as who will be providing those activities.

In a community setting, both the pharmacists and technicians will be involved. They do not have to be the only contact for students in this setting. Check with physicians who work closely with the pharmacy and see if students can spend some time in their offices. If the community setting is a chain store, include the district manager in the training functions. Many of the district managers are taking students full-time for courses, and they enjoy the opportunity to mentor students.

There are many other settings where students are trained: the pharmaceuti-

Do NOT

- Skimp on the time for orientation or eliminate what you believe are small things
- Say "Hey everyone, this is the student this month! Let me know if you need help."
- Tell students to help anyone who needs it
- Ignore covering student responsibilities
- Tell students you will worry about assignments as you go
- Provide students with only memorization activities
- Use students as free help

cal industry mail order companies, veterinary practice settings, home infusion services, and nursing homes. Various professionals and technical staff at each of these sites can become involved with student training.

Involving people in student training programs (especially people who often come into contact with students) is good practice, even if for logistical purposes only. The more people know about pharmacy education, the better students will be accepted, and the greater the chance for student success.

Continuous quality improvement should not be a scary process. It is a process that requires planning, integration of assessment, and a team effort. When putting together an experiential education training program, ask who will be involved, and how they will be involved before you start. Have a plan in place for training. Make sure that information on the program is both outgoing and incoming. Gather assessment often and from multiple sources. Learn from the information gathered and improve and build your program with each student you precept.

References

1. Accreditation Council for Pharmacy Education. Introduction to the professional degree program accreditation process. Available at: http://www.acpe-accredit.org/deans/accreditation.asp. Accessed May 2004.
2. American Society for Quality. American Society for Quality glossary. Available at: http://www.asq.org/info/glossary/c.html. Accessed May 2004.
3. Delaware Healthcare Association. Delaware Healthcare Association glossary of health care terms and acronyms. Available at: http://www.deha.org/Glossary/GlossaryC.htm. Accessed May 2004.
4. Mental Health Association. Available at: http//www.mh.state.oh.us. Accessed May 2004.

Continuous effort, not strength or intelligence, is the key to unlocking your potential.

Winston Churchill

Chapter 7

Partnerships with Schools

Lourdes M. Cuéllar, Sarah E. Lake-Wallace, Jennifer R. Myhra, Michael Piñón, Kevin Purcell

Chapter Outline

Every worthwhile accomplishment, big or little, has its stages of drudgery and triumph; a beginning, a struggle and a victory.

Mahatma Ghandi

Developing Partnerships–The School Perspective

Jennifer R. Myhra

Objective

- Clearly describe the role of the school or college of pharmacy, student intern, site, and preceptor.

Developing effective partnerships between academic institutions and practice facilities is one of the keys to creating a mutually beneficial, long-term and professionally rewarding experience for both entities. This relationship requires an initial buy-in on both sides that is achieved through an understanding of each other's goals, and then a nurturing of that relationship through constant two-way communication and feedback.

Academically based practice facilities, without question, understand the education of students as a primary mission along with care of patients. This is part of the culture of the facility, and the hospital administration must support an atmosphere through which this mission can be accomplished. Practice facilities outside of academic institutions, however, may or may not articulate student training as a part of their mission. Therefore, within the framework of that institution, it may be more difficult to provide the activities or personnel necessary to effectively teach and mentor students. The business of caring for patients may not be as easily integrated with the education of students even though the facility may desire to participate in such activities.

For colleges or schools of pharmacy, there are advantages of working with both academically based and nonacademic practice facilities. Educational institutions should recognize that each practice facility is unique, perhaps addressing health care specializations or patient populations that bring diversity to its inventory of practice experiences available to students. And, although it may seem more advantageous to work with an academic health facility, there are often not enough rotations within these entities to meet curricular needs.

Likewise, practice sites may be asked to work with one or more pharmacy schools in a geographic area. It is highly probable in these instances that the partnership between the facility and the educational institution is defined by different sets of goals, expectations, and written agreements set by that college's faculty and university governance, from one pharmacy program to the next. Although a minimum level of educational competence should be expected from students in any pharmacy program, some colleges or schools may place greater emphasis in one area than another. Thus, students are not a homogenous population as they proceed through the internship experiences.

How then, in consideration of the differences in practice facilities and academic institutions, is an effective partnership established? Roles, responsibilities, expectations, and mutual goals should be established, described in detail, and understood by all parties involved. Formal agreements should exist that define those general responsibilities and expectations that can be reduced to writing. The educational institution should have opportunities to give feedback to the practice facility and preceptor that are thoughtfully considered and acted on if otherwise appropriate. The site should give input to the college or school of pharmacy through invited membership on committees, internship program meetings, preceptor training, and other mechanisms. These will be described in the sections to follow.

Spectacular achievement is always preceded by unspectacular preparation.

Robert H. Schuller

Developing Partnerships—The Preceptor Perspective

Kevin Purcell

Objectives

- Learn to develop a true partnership between the preceptor's practice site and the school of pharmacy in order to assure success of the internship program for everyone.
- Understand the importance of continuous quality improvement once the internship is started.
- Document positive outcomes that affirm the value of the partnership and possibly justify the allocation of additional resources.

A true partnership must be developed between the preceptor's practice site and the school of pharmacy in order to assure success of the internship program for everyone. Partnership development takes time and effort but is critical to success. Time must be spent initially to learn the needs and expectations of each other. It is also important to understand the operation and culture of both organizations. The chances of building a successful long-term partnership are much greater if the site's practice model and the school's education and training program fit well together and the mission, vision, philosophy, and core values of both partners are in alignment.

A partnership may be defined by what is written on a piece of paper in the form of an educational affiliation agreement, but the success is determined by the relationships developed between key persons at the practice site and at the school of pharmacy. The preceptor in charge of coordinating the internship program at the site and the assistant/associate dean responsible for experiential education at the school need to work closely together and have periodic contact. This relationship is very important as the school administrator will be the site coordinator's primary contact person and interface with the school. Having a good relationship is especially important when trouble-shooting problems and dealing with difficult students.

A site visit should be scheduled so that the site coordinator and the school administrator can meet and begin forming their relationship. Information can be exchanged about the training opportunities at the site and the internship program requirements. Typically, schools will provide rotation-specific internship manuals that contain the goals and objectives, required learning activities and assignments, and evaluation form(s). The potential types of rotations and the number of preceptors available should be discussed, as well as the site capacity for students on a monthly and annual basis. This will be important when the site coordinator and school administrator work on constructing a schedule for student placement. Ultimately, a shared vision and plan for the future should be created. Then both site and school can budget for and allocate the necessary resources to accomplish mutual goals and objectives in a structured and timely manner. Future plans could include such things as slowly increasing the number of students per month, developing additional elective rotations, hiring more clinical pharmacists, recruiting and placing a faculty member(s) at the site, and developing or expanding residency programs at the site.

Although the educational affiliation agreement does not determine the success of the partnership, it is an important legal document as it defines the requirements for each partner. An educational affiliation agreement should be in place before students begin an internship at a practice site. This can be a time consuming process, especially if changes to the school's standard educational affiliation agreement are proposed either as a result of negotiation between the site coordinator and the school administrator or through review by the site's attorney. Of course, then the school's attorney must approve the proposed changes. Finally, people in each organization with the power to authorize such a partnership must sign the agreement. Both the practice site and the school will retain a copy for their records. Like any business transaction in which a written contract is made, do not rely on verbal commitments. For example, if the school has offered to pay the site for precepting services or to provide faculty appointments, textbooks, or library access to preceptors, that should be stated in the body of the text or in an appendix of the agreement. This can help prevent any misunderstanding and frustration from occurring later.

Preceptors should get actively involved as much as possible with the school and take advantage of any opportunities afforded. Attendance at annual statewide preceptor conferences or appreciation dinners can be fun and rewarding. Sometimes preceptor education programs are also offered at the local or regional level. Preceptors may be invited to faculty meetings, faculty development workshops, and faculty retreats. Preceptors may be asked to serve on an internship program advisory committee or preceptor advisory board. There is usually the opportunity to serve on a faculty committee (e.g., curriculum committee) if so desired. Preceptors can give lectures in courses or presentations to student professional organizations as well. These are all good ways to get involved, express your opinions and ideas, and interact more closely and frequently with students and fellow preceptors and faculty members.

Most pharmacists become preceptors to give something back to the profession. The intrinsic rewards are great. Serving as preceptor stimulates personal and professional growth and development and enhances professional satisfaction. Most preceptors also really enjoy teaching and helping others learn the art and science of pharmacy practice. In addition to all of this, there also may be some extrinsic benefits as well. Schools may pay practice sites or individual pharmacists for precepting services. Schools may also provide preceptors with faculty appointments, preceptor recognition certificates, school pins, library access, textbooks, journals, and free or discounted continuing pharmacy education. Schools may offer preceptors the chance to complete an advanced traineeship with a recognized faculty member at one of their best practice sites. Generally, teaching awards are presented to outstanding preceptors at an annual preceptor conference or awards ceremony. Hopefully, thank-you notes are periodically sent to preceptors to express the schools' gratitude for their services.

Once an internship program is started at a practice site, the process of continuous quality improvement (CQI) must begin. There are always opportunities for improvement and lessons to learn in order to become a better preceptor and build a better rotation. Obtaining student feedback on the preceptors and the practice site is critical to the CQI process. The school administrator should provide a summary of student evaluations of the site and the preceptors on a regular basis. This may be on an annual or semiannual basis depending on the numbers of students precepted during a given time period. It is important to assure the integrity of the evaluation process and maintain anonymity of comments if honest and useful information is to be obtained. Additionally, the preceptor can hold a debriefing session at the end of each rotation and obtain timely oral and/or written feedback from students for the purposes of CQI. Periodically the school administrator should make site visits. This allows the site coordinator the opportunity to seek his/her advice and for the school administrator to share information on best practices observed in other sites. Preceptors can also tell the school administrator their personal observations regarding student preparedness and assimilation of coursework and experiential competencies. Preceptors should also actively seek advice and share their ideas, successes, and failures with other preceptors they know.

Preceptors should share their innovations and success stories with their peers by making presentations at preceptor conferences, presenting posters at professional society meetings, and publishing articles in pharmacy journals. Positive outcomes may be documented that affirm the value of the partnership and possibly justify the allocation of additional resources. Improvements and desired increases may be measured in patient care, education, research, and administrative activities.

Example is not the main thing in influencing others. It is the only thing.

A. Schweitzer[1]

Roles of the Preceptor, School, Student, and Site

Michael Piñón

Objectives

- Learn to develop precepting methods to excel as a clinical instructor, an evaluator, and as a mentor.
- Determine the expectations of the preceptor with regard to administrative and teaching responsibilities.
- Integrate the roles of the student and the school to maximize precepting outcomes.

Role of the Preceptor

In both medical and pharmacy models, a substantial portion of the educational mission is superimposed on experiential training by preceptors. The preceptor is responsible for navigating and tailoring the students' educational experience, assessing student progression, and maintaining the physician-patient-pharmacist relationships within the patient care setting.

Pharmacy students observe and emulate their preceptor role models to develop their own standards and behaviors for future pharmacy practice. From aseptic technique to the conduct of patient interviews and physical assessments, students notice the nuances of their preceptor's behaviors toward patients, staff, and colleagues. Witnessing nonjudgmental interviewing and cultural competence, as well as the application of evidence-based medicine to patient problems, allows students to appreciate the importance of integrating the art and science of pharmacy in the delivery of high-quality patient care and will be further incorporated into the students' professional identity. Preceptors convey powerful messages that are typically not presented in the classroom.

While experiential rotations vary in the opportunity for hands-on experiences and in the number and quality of teacher-learner interactions, most students report that rotations offer closer supervision, greater exposure to a diversity of patient care issues, and more meaningful teacher-student interactions than are presented within the didactic classroom. Students often enter into longstanding relationships between themselves and their preceptors. Within the experiential setting, students learn by caring for patients in practice settings that have been created, cultivated, and nurtured by their preceptors. The experiences provided to students, and the willingness of institutional staff to include pharmacy students in patient care ongoing within these practice settings, are often representative of the professionalism of the preceptor and time he/she has committed to development of the practice site.

Introducing students to our profession can be one of the most satisfying experiences offered to a preceptor. Students have been waiting for several years to put into practice what they have learned in the classroom. They are often eager to begin their transition from students to health professionals. The responsibility and privilege of guiding students through this transition rests on the preceptor.

Preceptor self-assessment with regard to the mentoring of students should include:

- How does a preceptor demonstrate to students the importance of cultivating the pharmacist-patient relationship?
- How does a pharmacist respond to patient emotion, convey empathy, or motivate patients to change their behaviors?
- How does a pharmacist use knowledge of the unique qualities of the patient, family, and community to improve outcomes?
- How can a pharmacist manage time in a busy practice and balance his/her professional life?
- Is postgraduate training being encouraged?
- How can a pharmacist give back or contribute to the profession?

The Preceptor as a Clinical Instructor

Preceptors initiate students to a new and unfamiliar medical culture with particular customs, language, and procedures. Keep your clinical teaching simple. Students may not feel empowered to say no when they feel unprepared for a particular learning opportunity. Remembering your own early patient encounters may be of help in deciding what to emphasize and teach.

The Preceptor as an Evaluator

Students rely on their preceptors to provide feedback on their performance. When students are developing new skills, it is important to concentrate on providing specific positive feedback for work well done. Constructive feedback should be tailored to help students understand their learning needs. Students should understand that their rotation is an environment where they will learn by experience and inquiry. This will allow them to comfortably disclose uncertainties or learning needs.

The Preceptor as a Mentor

When students are assigned to any kind of experiential clerkship or rotation, particularly longitudinal clinical experience, preceptors have the opportunity to get to know them in depth. These kinds of relationships foster the opportunity to know students better than any other faculty member. You may be able to provide assistance as students formulate professional identities and goals. Being supportive during the difficult transition from the classroom to practice can help bolster students' much needed self-confidence. Enthusiasm for teaching and your professional practice is important in making your students' experience a positive one.

Expectations of the Preceptor

Administrative Responsibilities

- Orient students to the rotation and training site. Clearly identify specific service and personal expectations.
- Introduce to office and ancillary care staff and encourage them to be helpful and make students feel a part of the team.
- Complete a formal written evaluation of student performance during the rotation according to the school's policy.

- Contact the Regional Dean or Experiential Coordinator to discuss issues of concern and student performance.

Teaching Responsibilities

- Serve as a mentor who assists students in applying knowledge and building skills to perform assigned tasks and to problem-solve patient care.
- Provide appropriate training and supervision.
- Challenge students with deliberate and thoughtful questions.
- Allow students to participate in departmental or institutional activities.
- Provide written and verbal feedback to students in a constructive and timely manner.
- Be available, on site, for assistance during assigned tasks, training, and patient care activities.
- Share learning resources (texts, computers, and educational programs) sufficient to increase student knowledge and productivity.
- Assign readings, literature searches, or medical information gathering pertinent to patient care.
- Integrate students' didactic knowledge base into the designated or assigned pharmacy practice site.

Role of the School

The educational programs of the college work best when integrated with the pharmacy services of their affiliated heath care organizations. Routine visits by school representatives (Assistant or Associate Dean or Director of Experiential Education) to practice sites can prove valuable and can help build relationships between schools and their preceptors. These interactions allow school representatives to better understand practice site dynamics and issues, heighten awareness and understanding of students' clerkship rotation, and help the preceptors with continuous quality improvement of the clerkships. Student issues regarding their progress, expectations, evaluations, etc., should be addressed at this time. The school should seize every opportunity to establish, maintain, and improve good working relationships with both administrative and clinical staff at these sites.

Preceptors can give feedback to the school on training requirements and student preparation as well as on the organization and service provided to them by the school. This is also a great opportunity for the school representatives to provide preceptors with periodic summaries of students evaluations of them and their practice sites.

The performance of preceptors should be measured with established criteria. Individuals should be evaluated for the quality and effectiveness of their practice site, and also for the quality of their teaching and mentoring. The evaluation process should consider and acknowledge efforts of preceptor faculty that make contributions toward the advancement of the students' professional development, such as academic and postgraduate advising, career pathway counseling, research, and mentoring activities. Such evaluation criteria should consider not only student evaluations of the preceptor site, but also well-defined objective criteria for professional service, scholarship, and practice success.

Role of the Student

Experiential education is designed to help students become active participants in providing contemporary pharmaceutical care services. Under the direction of their preceptors, students will integrate their knowledge of pharmacotherapy, disease states, dosage formulations, and pharmacokinetics in developing and assessing therapeutic plans and evaluating drug selection for patients. Each rotation should emphasize outcomes-oriented decision making in clinical situations regarding drug therapy.

Students are expected to attend physician rounds, interdisciplinary team meetings, attend conferences and discussions, monitor and present assigned patients, and interact with patients and health care professionals. Over the course of their experience students will learn to develop recommendations and participate in decisions about drug therapy with regard to efficacy, toxicity, pharmacoeconomics, and unique methods of drug delivery.

At the end of each experiential rotation, students should be able to do the following:

- Dispense and compound prescriptions in accordance with all legal, ethical, and patient care standard practices.

- Prepare sterile and chemotherapeutic products in accordance with the accepted standard of practice.
- Apply case management skills to drug therapy selection, monitoring, and assessment.
- Develop a plan for continuity of care of patients for drug therapy as part of the health care team.
- Develop, implement, and document pharmaceutical care plans that manage patient care needs using drug monitoring and physical assessment skills.
- Identify barriers and propose solutions to manage common disease states in traditionally underserved populations with little or no access to the health care system.
- Use strategies to improve patient compliance with drug therapy regimens to enhance outcomes.
- Develop practice management skills relating to documentation and compensation issues, managed care, supervision of supportive or technical personnel, and administrative matters related to operations and patient outcomes.
- Demonstrate the ability to integrate distributive and clinical skills in providing pharmacist care.
- Actively participate in clinical process improvement activities and population based therapeutic drug decision making for targeted populations or groups of patients.
- Actively participate in activities related to health promotion and disease prevention in a variety of settings.

In addition, students will maximize their investment in education and the value of their experiential learning program by adhering to these guidelines:

- Contact the preceptor seven to ten days prior to the start of the rotation for the schedule, directions to the site, and any other pertinent information.
- Exhibit appropriate professional dress and behavior while on experiential learning assignments.
- Meet deadline established by the experiential learning office, coursemasters, and preceptors.

- Demonstrate an eagerness to increase knowledge, skills, and abilities through experiential learning.
- Make up any time away from the site for any reason (i.e., illness, religious/school/government holidays, school or personal activities, etc.) during the scheduled rotation dates.

Reference

1. Schweitzer A. *The World of Albert Schweitzer.* New York: Harper and Brothers; 1995.

We cannot discover new oceans until we have the courage to lose sight of the shore.

Muriel Chen

Educational Affiliation Agreements

Jennifer R. Myhra

Objective

- Discuss the contents of written agreements and how the language of various agreements affects all of the parties involved in the rotation experience.

Responsibilities of both the facility and the educational institution are reduced to writing and described in detail via the educational affiliation agreement. This agreement may originate with either party. If the college or school of pharmacy initiates an agreement and is part of a larger university or system of universities, the affiliation agreement may be standard for all health care-related schools, then defined for each individual program (i.e., pharmacy) via an amendment to the original educational affiliation. In the case where a site originates the affiliation agreement, it could be a standard agreement based with the facility's parent company or owner or it could be specific for the individual institution.

In any event, standard areas of responsibility that are addressed within these agreements usually include the following:

- Complete identification of both the educational facility and the practice site (full name, location, type of practice, affiliated institutions, etc.).
- Reference to the need for any additional amending agreements.
- Method(s) of conflict resolution.
- Responsibilities of the facility, including but not limited to the following:
  1. Compliance with all applicable state, federal, and municipal laws, rules and regulations, and with all applicable requirements of accreditation authorities.
  2. Permission for a designated university representative to inspect the facilities for the purpose of the educational experience.

3. Appropriate supervision of students by a qualified practitioner and that practitioner's appointment or other recognition within the university.
4. Designating a liaison from the facility to the college or school of pharmacy.
5. Providing appropriate space for student activities.
6. Providing equipment, supplies, qualified personnel, and supervised access to patients required for educational activities.
7. Maintaining of all required licenses.
8. Providing an orientation to the facility.
9. Assuming sole responsibility for patient care.

- Responsibilities of the educational institution, including but not limited to the following:
  1. Providing the facility with names of the students assigned to the facility.
  2. Assigning to the facility only those students who have completed the prerequisites for participation.
  3. Designating a university liaison to the facility.
  4. Developing criteria for student evaluation and grading.
  5. Requiring students to carry professional liability insurance.
  6. Removing a student from the facility when the student has engaged in professional misconduct as defined within the agreement (e.g., student compromises patient safety or discloses confidential patient information).
  7. Compliance with accreditation standards.
  8. Periodic review of the program.
  9. Ensuring that students are registered, if appropriate, under state law, as interns.

- Term of agreement and effective date.
- Indemnification of either party.
- General provisions, including but not limited to the following:
  1. Statement that students are in the pharmacy program and not employees.
  2. Student responsibility for transportation and meals.

3. Nondiscrimination clause.
4. Privacy statement(s).

Language that requires the educational institution to guarantee good student mental and physical health is controversial with many universities because of student privacy and disability issues. Additionally, educational institutions cannot guarantee that students will behave professionally or be highly motivated; however, it is imperative to articulate in writing the sequence of events within both the site and the school that are necessitated by unprofessional conduct.

In addition to these items, agreement regarding payment to the facility or preceptor for student rotations may be included. Alternatively, this can be handled through service contracts.

◆ **Preceptor Pearls**

- Become thoroughly familiar with the responsibilities of both the facility and the educational institution as articulated in any formal written agreements.
- Make sure that those responsible for establishing affiliation agreements within your facility begin the process well ahead of when you are expecting students in the facility.

The rush to amend existing affiliation agreements and put in place new ones was precipitated by the implementation of HIPAA in 2003. Additionally, this process is constantly fueled by a need for corporations, facilities, and/or universities to include language in all formal written agreements that works, to the extent possible, to avoid litigation from other parties. Add to this the fact that various groups and/or individuals and/or departments within the facility may be involved in the review of contracts. All of these factors combined result in agreements that take months to even years to finalize between contractual parties. This can ultimately delay the assignment of students to a facility.

Knowing is not enough; we must apply. Willing is not enough; we must do.

Johann Wolfgang von Goethe

Benefits for Preceptors

Michael Piñón, Lourdes M. Cuéllar, Kevin Purcell

Objectives

- Describe the importance of external reward systems that help acknowledge and recognize the efforts of preceptors by schools of pharmacy.
- Identify methods of providing acknowledgement and recognition to preceptors.
- Discuss how external rewards can develop and nurture relationships among preceptors, practice sites, and schools of pharmacy.

In 1995, The American College of Clinical Pharmacy published in Pharmacotherapy, *Rewards and Advancements for Clinical Pharmacy Practitioners.*[1] Within this paper, Dr. Zarowitz describes pharmacy practitioners as having a "fundamental need to be noticed, to feel important, and to be recognized for excellence."[1] Although participating in a student's progress can provide gratification that may be sufficient for many preceptors, external reward systems, awarded by the schools of pharmacy, that are designed to recognize pharmacy practitioners are necessary and in many instances lacking.

Faculty Appointments and Promotion

The awarding and designation of formal adjunct faculty appointments to medical practitioners has been widely adopted and recognized by medical schools. These titles and awards demonstrate a sincere effort by medical academia to distinguished deserving and dedicated practitioners that have committed their time as preceptors and as mentors to the school's students. Additionally, such awards provide an incentive for preceptors to become involved and committed with the school and to establish new or maintain existing clerkships for students.

The American Council on Pharmaceutical Education (ACPE) is expanding the requirement for Doctor of Pharmacy degree programs to include both early and late experiential education. As a result, preceptors are becoming an increasingly more important part of the pharmacy school faculty. Many highly educated and trained preceptors should be considered to receive a clinical faculty appointment or adjunct clinical faculty appointment. This not only provides them some formal recognition, but also makes them feel more of a part of the school and faculty. Use of titles such as "practitioner faculty," "preceptor faculty," or "volunteer faculty" does not convey the same message or meaning and contributes to the creation of a perceived class or caste system between full-time faculty members and preceptors.

Objective and rational criteria should be in place for the equitable awarding clinical faculty appointments (e.g., clinical instructor, clinical assistant professor, etc.) or adjunct clinical faculty appointments (e.g., adjunct clinical assistant professor, adjunct clinical associate professor) to preceptors. Additionally, criteria and a process should also be in place so preceptors who make outstanding accomplishments (in pharmacy practice, education, research and scholarly activity, and service to the school, community, or profession) can apply for non-tenure track promotion.

All preceptors should be given the opportunity to receive faculty appointments. Preceptors who make these types of accomplishments will be more valuable to the school and are worthy of recognition through promotion. Also, if preceptors have an academic appointment, they will usually list it in addition to their institutional affiliations on any presentations they make or papers they publish, which can bring additional recognition to the schools.

Preceptor Development

Preceptors want to improve their teaching and mentoring abilities. Effective teaching requires knowledge of the discipline, effective communication skills, and an understanding of student challenges and capabilities. It is imperative to have practice faculty who are role models for professional attributes and behaviors so as to effectively mentor, monitor, and evaluate students. These role models should also be responsive and sensitive to cultural and ethnic differences in student practice settings.

Having regularly scheduled, live preceptor education programs, both general and rotation-specific, are very useful and desired by preceptors. These programs could involve educational technologies and techniques that support various modes of educational delivery, such as simulations, case studies, evaluation, and clinical performance assessments. Another valuable venue for preceptor development is formal or informal round table discussions that can be held during professional organizations' annual meetings. Preceptors can network and discuss issues pertinent to their continuing development as effective educators and mentors.

Additionally, web-based self-study modules on various aspects of teaching would also be well-received by those who cannot attend the live sessions. For preceptors who are trying to improve their patient care skills, the opportunity to apply for an advanced clinical traineeship with a distinguished faculty member could be a great learning experience. The short, intensive training provided would ultimately improve both the preceptors' clinical practice and the rotations offered to students.

Scholarship and Resources for Education or Research

Academic faculty members have the responsibility to generate and disseminate knowledge through scholarship; preceptors should be encouraged to participate in the area of scholarship as well. Accomplishment in this area can be demonstrated by productive research and scholarly activities such as contributions to the scientific, professional, and educational literature, publication of books and review articles, as well as involvement of pharmacy students in the research and publication process.

Fostering an environment that encourages scholarly contributions by preceptors contributes to the advancement of knowledge and intellectual growth of students in experiential rotations. Furthermore, schools should encourage affiliations and foster relationships with institutions that provide postgraduate residency and fellowship programs. Library and educational resources are essential tools that support clinical pharmacy services utilized by both preceptors and students. These resources often support research and scholarly activities in accord with the mission of the school. There may be resources that the schools can make available to preceptors. Access to journals via library collections or online services, interlibrary loans, and technologies should meet the needs of preceptors and students alike at experiential practice sites. Providing key textbooks or journals to support specific rotations at practice sites would also be beneficial.

Support for Professional Enhancement

The establishment of a professional enhancement fund could be accessed by preceptors for travel to professional meetings, attendance at seminars designed to enhance their professional knowledge or skills, or to represent the school in a public forum.

Involvement of Preceptors in School Activities and Functions

Preceptors should be encouraged to be involved as much as possible in school activities and functions. This not only enhances their understanding of the educational programs and the expectations of clinical faculty members, but also garners loyalty and better integrates them into the school culture. Including preceptors on the school list can keep them informed and up-to-date. Preceptors could be invited to participate in faculty meetings, faculty retreats, and faculty workshops. If the school conducts journal club activities or grand rounds, preceptors should be invited to attend and actively participate.

Additionally, preceptors could be invited to serve on faculty committees or to give guest lectures. Preceptors should be invited to attend the graduation and awards ceremonies as they have developed relationships with and helped in the education and training of the graduating students and residents. Preceptors appreciate being sent a calendar of school events or at least a link to the place on the school website where it is posted. Preceptors should also receive copies of the school newsletter, journal, and annual reports so they can stay in touch with what is going on at the school.

Compensation and Gifts-in-Kind

Preceptors realize that school resources are limited. Some schools compensate preceptors or the health system financially in return for precepting students. This is generally specified contractually in the form of affiliation agreements between the practice site and the school.

While it may be difficult and intangible to establish the true cost of precepting students, the absolute value is priceless. Any fees the schools pay for precepting services are very much appreciated by preceptors. Such compensation has several benefits such as financing travel and expenses to professional meetings or educational resources needed by the preceptor or institution such as books, software, and supplies.

However, schools should have clearly stated policies on financial compensation for preceptor services. Whether or not a school decides to compensate, it should do so equitably and consistently among all preceptors or institutions. Funding should be free of restrictions that may interfere with sound educational and ethical policies. Criteria developed should be used in a manner that maintains the integrity and supports the mission of the school.

Forming an advisory board of preceptors from various practice settings and regions to assist schools in setting policies consistent with school budgets and in communicating the policies and rationale to other preceptors should be considered.

In lieu of financial compensation, there may be other gifts-in-kind that schools can provide to preceptors. Preceptors do like to receive school pins, and they wear them with pride. Uniforms such as scrubs or lab coats with school logos may also be appropriate. Discounts for continuing education programs offered by the schools would be appreciated and could also promote professional growth and development of preceptors. Many preceptors are very loyal to the schools, especially if they are alumni, and discounts on clothing or other memorabilia from the schools would be well-received. As members of the faculty, preceptors may also be considered having benefits such as access to faculty parking, gymnasium, or recreational facilities, and discounts to collegiate sporting or fine art events.

Preceptor Awards and Appreciation Dinners or Conferences

Preceptors of the Year awards are cherished and there can never be too many awards given. These awards can include preceptors in different practice settings (e.g., hospital or health system, community, etc.), in different training regions, and for all the student classes (second-, third-, and fourth-professional years). Notifying the preceptor's manager or supervisor and the company president or hospital CEO of the award provides further recognition. Additionally, local papers often have a section for publishing short press releases related to promotions and awards received by citizens of the community. Other innovative preceptor awards could also be developed so that more than a small handful of the hundreds of preceptors per school are recognized each year. Preceptors are very thankful for and truly enjoy annual preceptor appreciation dinners and conferences. These functions are ideal settings at which to recognize preceptors in front of their peers. The group discussions and educational programming are well-received and also facilitate professional growth and development of preceptors as clinical faculty members.

Recognition of Preceptors' Accomplishments in School Publications

Often schools publish an annual report. Among other things, the annual reports usually recognize the accomplishments of full-time faculty members (e.g., presentations, publications, grants, awards, elected/appointed positions, etc.). Some preceptors make significant contributions in these areas as well. Schools should utilize this opportunity to recognize their preceptors' accomplishments along with those of full-time faculty members in the annual report or other school publications. Preceptors are faculty members too and want to be recognized for their contributions to the schools.

Personal Letters of Appreciation

Preceptors enjoy being recognized for their service to the schools. Publishing the names of preceptors and formally thanking them in both school and professional society newsletters and journals (hard copy and electronic editions) is recommended. Sending individual thank-you letters to preceptors with an inspiring message at the end of the academic year has extra meaning. Making handwritten comments in the letter to outstanding preceptors is truly meaningful and enhances their desire and commitment to become even better preceptors. Preceptors appreciate the extra time and effort it takes to do this, especially for schools with hundreds of preceptors. Invitations to school activities, such as student presentations or grand rounds, receptions, picnics, fundraisers, faculty outings and retreats, journal clubs, lectures, etc., can help build camaraderie and unity between school faculty and preceptors.

Summary

Preceptors would like to develop relationships and partnerships with pharmacy schools that benefit their practice sites, the schools, the students, and themselves. Preceptors want to be valued members of the faculty team. Although the list of ideas for ways to recognize and reward preceptors is not meant to be exhaustive, implementing some of these ideas along with other creative reward mechanisms can help build camaraderie, unity, communication, and respect between full-time faculty members and preceptors. More importantly, it will make preceptors feel good about themselves and the jobs they are doing.

Reference

1. Zarowitz B. Rewards and advancements for clinical pharmacy practitioners. *Pharmacotherapy*. 1995;15(1):99–105.

Who dares wins.

British Special Air Service (SAS) motto

Benefits for Site

Jennifer R. Myhra

Objectives

- Articulate both the intrinsic and extrinsic benefits for the preceptor.
- Describe the benefits to the practice site.

It would be difficult for practice facilities to participate in student education and training unless tangible benefits are apparent to the pharmacy practice facility. Indeed, the labor-intensive activities involved with hosting students on rotations should come with some type of reward. Each site will identify these benefits in ways appropriate to the practice setting, and educational institutions will provide these based on their means.

Benefits can be monetary, "in kind," or nonmonetary. Monetary remuneration, in the form of payment for student rotations or partial or full salary for cofunded pharmacist staff/faculty preceptors, is a type of arrangement that can be made between the practice facility and the educational institution. In-kind benefits can include access by the facility to university resources not otherwise available such as online libraries and databases, or access of the site to software, computers, reference books, educational programming, and other resources at reduced or no cost.

What do pharmacy administrators define as those nonmonetary, sometimes intrinsic, benefits to the site? A select group of pharmacy administrators questioned on this topic has provided the following perspectives on the advantages of participating in pharmacy student education:

- Assists in recruiting future pharmacist employees. In geographic areas of critical shortage, this is described as one of the top advantages to hosting students.
- Shortens training time for possible future employees.

- Contributes to the educational mission of the facility.
- Increases pharmacy visibility/presence in patient care areas of the facility.
- Provides professional development of staff preceptors.
- Exposes students to the concept of advanced training (residencies).
- Helps to maintain relationships with educational institutions in areas outside of the internship, such as research.
- Gains personal satisfaction by serving as teachers and mentors to future pharmacists.

The students themselves benefit the site in the following ways:

- They are a good resource for special projects to which staff can devote little time, and similarly they often help distribute the workload of an individual preceptor so he/she can do more when students are present in the facility.
- Students help keep pharmacy staff current in asking questions and students prompt institutions to review practices that may need updating.

Therefore, within the array of tangible and nontangible advantages described above, it should be possible to determine benefits to the site that either the facility can recognize on its own, and/or that can be provided by the college or school of pharmacy.

Obstacles don't have to stop you. If you run into a wall, don't turn around or give up. Figure out how to climb it, go through it, or work around it.

Michael Jordan

Ways to Become a Better Preceptor

Jennifer R. Myhra

Objectives

- Recognize and participate in those activities that will make you a better preceptor.
- Provide feedback to the school regarding student preparedness and educational outcomes.

Becoming a better preceptor is a continuous quality improvement process. Initial expectations can be established by the educational institution up front and appropriate training provided. However, there is nothing like supervising individual students on rotation to help you identify your weaknesses and build your strengths.

How does one rate oneself as a baseline? Verbal feedback from students is one method. The questions can be simple: "How am I doing as your preceptor?" or "Are there things that I can do differently to be a better preceptor to you?" or "What was your favorite thing about this rotation, and what was your least favorite?" Individual students have specific needs and may give different answers of varying length and detail. At least with direct questioning you are providing an opportunity for students to give direct answers, and every bit of information helps. Granted, there may be some students that fear retribution of some type and may hesitate for one reason or another to be forthright, but most of the feedback you receive via this type of questioning will likely be of some benefit.

Additionally, feedback from the college or school that students provide through formal evaluation processes, which is then shared with the preceptor, can be extremely helpful. Rules within academic institutions may vary in terms of sharing the information provided by students as a part of this process, but hopefully it can occur. This evaluative process may include questions related to activities and outcomes of the rotation experience itself that reflect on the involvement of the preceptor in the experience. Specific to the individual preceptor, questions asked could focus on the following:

- Preparation for the internship
- Enthusiasm for the experience
- Expectations for the experience as communicated to the student
- Acessibility
- Willingness to answer questions
- Quality and quantity of feedback during the experience
- Degree of supervision
- Role as a mentor

Participating in preceptor education and training programs offered by colleges or schools of pharmacy or professional associations also helps preceptors fine-tune their teaching and mentoring skills. There is no question that continuing education programs focusing on therapeutics helps create better preceptors by continually developing contemporary pharmacists. However, those programs focusing on the uniqueness of the preceptor-student relationship are extremely beneficial in developing effective teachers and mentors.

> **◆ PRECEPTOR PEARLS**
>
> - Talk with interns regularly to ensure that you and the students have a mutual understanding of expectations for the rotation experience.
> - Take advantage of educational opportunities that train you how to be a good teacher, mentor, and evaluator of student performance.

A willingness to "give back" to the profession and/or educational institution from which you graduated or with which you are affiliated, as well as being amenable to the regular assignment of pharmacy students to your practice site, goes a long way in sustaining the qualities seen in an effective preceptor. However, it is important to take advantage of educational and training opportunities to not only further refine precepting skills, but also to maintain a high level of enthusiasm for your critical role in this process that is contagious throughout your professional life.

I know of no more encouraging fact than the unquestionable ability of man to elevate his life by conscious effort.

Henry David Thoreau

Providing Feedback to Schools on Student Preparedness and Assimilation of Didactic and Practice Competencies

Sarah E. Lake-Wallace

Objectives

- Establish the basic needs of the school.
- Understand the importance of expectations.
- Determine how to partner with the school to address difficult students.
- Address failing a student.
- Basic needs of schools.

Previous chapters have discussed the need for effective communication and effective evaluations. These same skills are just as essential in providing feedback to the schools. Hopefully most of the time, you will only give positive feedback to the school, but it is just as important to be honest about problems and issues.

The first step in this process is to establish who are the appropriate contacts and the best methods for communicating with that individual. In developing the initial relationship with the school, ask who is responsible for scheduling the students and who handles performance issues. Contact these individuals before there are any issues in order to help establish a relationship that can be useful in problem solving.

Another important area is to keep up with the required paperwork (evaluations, timesheets, etc.). Schools are usually required to maintain these basic forms to meet accreditation and regulatory standards. By keeping up your end of the responsibility, you can establish a common ground of respect.

Help schools plan their schedules by advising them of the dates you will not be available at your work site. It is useful for the school to know if the student is going to have to be in different locations due to a preceptor's vacation or illness. This information allows the school to locate the student if needed. As soon as you are aware of workflow or staffing changes that will affect your site's ability to take students, you should let the school know. Schedules do change, but advance notice allows the school to find alternative sites or adjust times. If you change your work site, inform the school of this as well. Developing a good relationship with quality preceptors can be difficult. Many schools want to maintain the relationship not only with the site, but also with the individual. The relationship between school and preceptor is important, but for it to be an effective relationship, you must keep an open line of communication.[1]

Establishing Expectations

At the same time, you should establish your expectations of the school. They should be told how far in advance you need a schedule of students. Let them know if your site requires any specific paperwork to be completed before students arrive on site. Let them know if there are times that you are not able to take students due to vacations or workload. Tell them the best way to contact you.

The school usually provides basic goals for rotations. You should use these as a baseline for creating your expectations of the students. You should communicate these to the students and use them as a basis of your evaluation. By establishing your expectations with the students, it may help avoid misunderstandings and give them specific goals to work toward. If there are problems with the students, you should also share your expectations with the school so they can understand your point of reference.

Sharing Evaluations

The next level of communication should include honest evaluations about student performance. You should try to be as objective as possible and try to limit the influence of personality differences. It can be helpful to review the specific goals of the rotation and relate comments back to these. Lickert scales on student skills may be an efficient manner of evaluation, but written comments make it possible to develop a full picture of strengths and weaknesses. Written comments not only improve student understanding of strengths, but also help the school compare activities and skills between rotations.

As with most effective relationships, the communication between schools and preceptors should start early and occur often. Just as you would not want to find out five minutes before a meeting that the materials were not prepared, schools cannot make necessary changes if they are told at the end of a rotation that students did not meet the minimum requirements. If you are having problems with a student, notify the appropriate individuals as early in the rotation as possible. If in the first weeks of a rotation, a student is not meeting expectation, this should be expressed to the school no later than the midpoint of the rotation. This allows time to address specific problems and create a plan to improve the student's outcome. If a student cannot eventually make up the difference, and it is necessary to give a failing grade, the school is now also prepared to make additional plans. Informing the school of the problems you experienced with a student allows the school to put together the entire picture if the student protests the grade.

If a student is having difficulty in the experience, consider the following issues:

- Is there a problem integrating knowledge with clinical decisions?
- Is it a communication problem?
- Is there difficulty working effectively with physicians, nurses, or other health care providers?

These issues can be difficult to overcome, but it is essential for schools to know about these crucial skills. If a student is having problems with these issues with you as a preceptor, these same problems may continue on other rotations if they are not addressed.

Working with Problem Students

Neither a preceptor nor a school wants to see students fail. All efforts should be taken to identify the barriers to success. The first step is, of course, to discuss these issues with students while keeping the school aware of your concerns. The next step is to get the school involved in problem solving. When working with a student that does not meet the minimum requirement, work with the school to develop a plan for improvement. This plan could include moving the student off site until issues can be resolved, assigning additional reading, or providing additional time on a rotation.[2] If these interventions still do not allow the student to progress, and failing the student is necessary, document the actions taken to help the student. The school also needs specific details on how the student failed to meet expectations. Just as most employees have a superior to report to, within a school system if a student appeals a failure, he or she can appeal. The school cannot accurately represent its side without details. Documentation of all details is important, including concerns about work problems such as tardiness.

When examining the barriers to success, consider personality issues, cultural issues, personal issues, and lack of knowledge. These problems can make for a difficult preceptor-student relationship, but by specifically addressing them, it may be possible for the student to succeed in the experience. Schools often have experience resolving these issues and can serve as resource for preceptors.

Personality issues may not be able to be resolved, but a working relationship is possible. Though it would be nice to be friends with your student, your primary goal and responsibility is to facilitate learning.

Today's students come from a wide variety of backgrounds and cultures. Cultural issues can effect how a student addresses superiors or approaches projects. Addressing cultural issues can help establish each person's expectations and avoid misconceptions.

Personal issues can include changes in dietary or exercise habits, complicated emotional relationships, or just the inability to manage all the changes during rotations. It is not necessarily appropriate to try to solve a student's personal issues, but it is important for the student to know how personal issues are affecting his or her performance. It may be important to help the student find outside help, and the schools often have resources in this area as well. This is also a good opportunity to reestablish your expectations.

Finally, if a student has knowledge deficits, it may be possible to assign additional readings or tutorial time. If you have discovered a significant knowledge deficit that affects a student's performance, the school may have resources to help address the problems as well.[3]

Failing Students

On the other side, the school is not a dumping ground for personality differences or students who do not fill the usual mold. It is unreasonable to assume the school has some magical method to solve all problems. Difficult students cannot always be moved from the site. Schools struggle with how to motivate students just as preceptors do. The schools should be viewed and treated as a partner in developing students into practitioners.

You also should not assume that the school will take care of a problem you do not want to address. If you do not fairly evaluate a student because you do not want to deal with the emotional side of failing a student, the school has no grounds on which to fail a student. Failing a student is hopefully a rare event, but you should always consider the impact the student will have on the profession and future patients. The decision to fail a student should not be taken lightly and will never be an easy experience. Failing a student may give that person the opportunity to become a better practitioner. Remember, if the student does not meet expectations, it is the student who caused the failure, not you. This relates back to the importance of establishing your expectations early and using these as the focus of your evaluation.

Make sure all steps taken to address deficiencies are documented. Let the school know you are intending to fail a student and what this decision is based on. Explain to the student how this decision was reached and how it can be avoided in the future.

Conclusion

The schools of pharmacy are partners with preceptors in developing future practitioners, and they should be treated as such. The experiential year of training is just as essential as all other formalized training pharmacy students complete. Colleges of pharmacy try to find the best faculty to instruct students during the didactic training; they also try to find the best instructors for the experiential year—the preceptors. As such, they depend on the preceptors to

◆ Preceptor Pearls

- Communicate regularly about problems and needs.
- Use the school as a problem-solving resource.
- Do not wait until the end of a rotation to bring serious problems to the school's attention.
- Try to determine what the barriers are to success and develop plans to overcome them.
- If you have come to the difficult decision to fail a student, work with the school to document appropriately the actions and activities that led to this outcome.

provide truthful evaluations of student skills and judge their ability to be pharmacy practitioners. Preceptors have the unique opportunity to work one-on-one with students and thoroughly evaluate their skills. The schools are dependent on preceptors to share this information.

References

1. Woo M. [e-mail]. University of Houston, College of Pharmacy; June 9, 2004.
2. Sayer M, Chaput De Saintonge M, Evans D, et al. Support for students with academic difficulties. *Med Educ.* 2002;36(7):643–50.
3. Kleffner JH, Hendrickson WD. Effective clinical teaching. December 2001 Available at: http://www.utexas.edu/pharmacy/general/experiential/practitioner/edopps.html. Accessed June 9, 2004.

It is from numberless diverse acts of courage and belief that human history is shaped. Each time a man stands up for an ideal, or acts to improve the lot of others, or strikes out against injustice, he sends forth a tiny ripple of hope.

Robert F. Kennedy

Chapter 8

Teaching Students about Cultural, Social, and Economic Issues Relating to Health Care

Lourdes M. Cuéllar, Nicanora C. Cuéllar

Chapter Outline

There is incredible liberation in realizing you can change the world simply by changing your perception.

Deepak Chopra, MD

Effectively Educating and Precepting a Diverse Student Population

Lourdes M. Cuéllar

Objectives

- Define diversity.
- Demonstrate the value of the diversity of our student population.
- Recognize our own biases or stereotypes and how they impact our ability to be effective preceptors.

In the book *Building a House for Diversity,*[1] R. Roosevelt Thomas, Jr. states that although race and ethnicity are the most obvious components of culture, there are many factors that shape a person's values, ideas, attitudes, and experiences. These include age, gender, disability, sexual orientation, level of education, income, preferred language, urban versus rural location, native versus foreign-born status, and customs, beliefs, and practices. An appreciation of the diversity of our students by health care organizations and preceptors is especially important today as health-systems and health care practitioners must respond to an increasing racially and ethnically diverse patient population.

A quick review of the demographic statistics of today's pharmacy students indicate that the portrait of our future practitioners differs significantly than what it was even 10 years ago. The scales have tilted with regard to gender (far more females) and education, with many schools admitting students (in some cases greater than 30%) with prior degrees, including advanced degrees. In addition many of the current students are older than the average college student. Likewise, the cultural or ethnic diversity of pharmacy students is significant in many areas of the U.S. However, the diversity of our pharmacy graduates does not match the growing diverse demographics of the U.S. population. The chance of the composition of the health care workforce in the

U.S. reflecting the diversity of our population in the near future is low.

Roosevelt[2] indicates that in the U.S. diversity has been addressed from several different perspectives:

- Civil rights—which seeks to end discrimination and racism and to comply with legal requirements.
- Women's rights—which focuses on eliminating sexism.
- Humanitarianism—which seeks to foster good relations through enhanced tolerance, acceptance, and understanding of individual differences.
- Moral responsibility—when individuals seek to live their moral beliefs by doing the "right thing."
- Social responsibility—where the objective is to be a good corporate citizen.

These perspectives are all different, and they are all equally legitimate. Today, organizational focus has turned toward cultural awareness or valuing differences.

The Institute of Medicine's (IOM) report, *In the Nation's Compelling Interest: Ensuring Diversity in the Health Care Workforce*[3] states that increasing racial and ethnic diversity among health care professionals is a very important aspect of providing health care because evidence suggests that diversity is associated with improved access to care for racial and ethnic minorities. In addition, it provides for greater patient choice in providers, improved patient satisfaction, better patient-clinician communication, and better educational experiences for health profession students.

Preceptors should be aware that culture greatly influences how students view their world while at school, home, or on experiential rotation. Some areas where cultural differences exist include the generally accepted roles for women and men; the importance of the individual versus the family or community; the role of religion in everyday life; body language; personal interactions; and boundaries regarding eye contact and personal space. It also affects how students may deal with critically ill patients and death. Students often bring with them their own history or beliefs regarding folk wisdom and common sense compared to formal education and scientific knowledge. The preceptor should thoughtfully inquire about student beliefs regarding illness versus wellness and holistic approach to health (mind, body, spirit) versus western medicine. As we move further toward evidence-based medicine, the need for alternative thera-

◆ Preceptor Pearls

- Become acquainted with your students individually; try to understand their interests, beliefs, and values. Do this on Day One.
- Learn every student's name and the name he/she prefers to be called by, and use that name. If you are not sure, ask for the correct pronunciation.
- Try to anticipate and acknowledge issues of sexuality, religion, or other values when you give projects or assignments.
- Introduce controversial topics in impersonal or nonjudgmental ways.
- Balance practical problem-solving techniques with fundamental methods.
- Do not overlook capable but quiet students; give male and female students equal attention when mentoring and when providing feedback.
- Treat students as individuals not as representatives of their gender or ethnicity.
- Do not assume that there is a collective identity minority students share.
- Do not make assumptions regarding a student's language capabilities based on ethnic background. (e.g., a student with a Hispanic last name may not necessarily read, speak, or understand Spanish).

(continued, page 229)

pies and their benefits will go under even greater scrutiny and potentially could be ignored or dismissed. Consequently, there will be even further potential for conflict relating to culture and its role in patient care, making an understanding of cultural diversity even more important.

Preceptors should recognize their own biases or stereotypes. Do you interact with students in ways that manifest double standards? Do you undervalue comments made by students whose English is accented or who appear foreign? Preceptors need to acknowledge and accept that cultural differences exist and it impacts their interaction with students. It is important to understand that incorporating the strengths of many cultures enhances the ca-

- Do not assume all students are heterosexual; respond firmly to inappropriate remarks.
- Take advantage of life experiences as well as the different perspectives that older students bring to the experiential rotation.
- Remember that older students may be dealing with children, mortgages, jobs, marriages, or divorces while they study to become a pharmacist.
- Assume that students hold different religious beliefs. Accommodate students' important religious holidays. Allow for them in planning the student schedule.
- If you have a student with a physical disability or challenge, ask the student privately if there is anything you can do to facilitate learning. Adapt to the student's need without lowering your usual course standards.
- Assume that certain topics may affect some students personally, for example, dealing with illness and disease.
- Monitor your own behavior in responding to students.
- Remember you teach what you are! Your training style reflects your knowledge, interests, and beliefs.

pacity of the whole group. Likewise, the preceptor should recognize that diversity *within* cultures is as important as diversity *between* cultures.

As preceptors and educators we need to value diversity. It is very important to avoid ethnocentrism where we believe our own culture is the best and the only way of doing things. The most important concept to keep in mind is that teaching for diversity means teaching to each *individual*. One of the greatest challenges you face is accommodating your teaching or precepting in a way that will meet the different learning styles of each student. By taking an interest in the students' experiences, interests, beliefs, and goals, you take the most important step in making the students feel that they will succeed on your rotation.

Remember as a preceptor you are a role model to your students. Share you own experiences and process of developing awareness of gender, recognition of sexual orientation, race, and ethnic stereotypes and issues. Help students understand the value of a diverse perspective in their future professional lives. Use examples from your own life and practice.

Health care practitioners need to learn the value of a culturally diverse environment, experience culture and gender differences, and appreciate the value of diversity in their daily decision-making process. Teach students the importance of integrating values and beliefs into the daily operations of their practice. Preceptors can exemplify this cultural awareness in their daily practice while interacting with their colleagues, other health care providers, and patients. This is integral to the cultural proficiency process. Reach out to students who are different in race, culture, or gender. Teach all students how to navigate successfully within a diverse population.

References

1. Thomas, RR. *Building a House for Diversity*. New York: AMACOM Publishers; 1999.
2. Thomas, RR. *Beyond Race and Gender: Unleashing the Power of Your Total Work Force by Managing Diversity.* New York: AMACOM Publishers; 1991.
3. Institute of Medicine (IOM). *The Nation's Compelling Interest: Ensuring Diversity in the Health Care Workforce*. Washington, DC: National Academy Press; 2004.

The ultimate measure of a man is not where he stands in moments of comfort and convenience, but where he stands at times of challenge and controversy.

Martin Luther King, Jr.

Health Disparities: What Pharmacy Students Need to Know

Lourdes M. Cuéllar

Objectives

- Define health disparities.
- Delineate disease states where disparities exist in specific racial or ethnic populations.
- Identify factors that contribute to health disparities.

The National Institutes of Health define health disparity as differences in the incidence, prevalence, mortality, and burden of diseases and other adverse health conditions that exist among specific populations groups in the United States. Recent studies and reports imply that there are differences not only in the services received by racial and ethnic minorities and people of lower socio-economic status, but also in the quality of those services. These racial and ethnic minority groups include African Americans, American Indians, Alaska Natives, Asian Americans, Hispanic Americans, and Pacific Islanders. The consistencies of the research findings were quite notable.

While death rates from breast cancer have declined during the 1990s, they remain higher among African American women. Women of racial and ethnic minorities are also less likely to receive Pap tests that can detect precancerous changes in the cervix and could prevent cervical cancer. Death rates from cardiovascular diseases are about 30% higher among African Americans. In March 2002, The Institute of Medicine (IOM) published its report, *Unequal Treatment: Confronting Racial and Ethnic Disparities in Healthcare.*[1] The IOM study committee found that health disparities exist in a number of areas including cardiovascular disease, HIV/AIDS, diabetes, cancer, mental illness and in routine treatments for common health problems.

There are numerous factors that contribute to health care disparities. These include cultural and language barriers (e.g., the provider not understanding the health beliefs or health seeking behaviors of their patients) and the lack of interpretative services for patients with limited or lack of English proficiency. Other factors include the patients' inability to access care, utilize services, and navigate health care systems; economic factors (inability to pay, including lack of health insurance); where many minorities go to receive care (less likely to access care in a private physician's office); the cultural competency of the health care provider; and patients' general health literacy.

In addition, there are factors identified by the IOM report that relate specifically to the patients' encounters with health care providers that may contribute to health disparities. These include the providers' real or perceived bias against minority patients, and stereotypes held by the providers about their patients' behaviors (e.g., response to pain) or health of a particular minority group (e.g., obesity). There is considerable empirical evidence that even well-intentioned non-Hispanic whites—who are not overtly biased and who do not believe that they are prejudiced—typically demonstrate unconscious implicit negative racial attitudes and stereotypes.[1]

For many racial and ethnic minorities in the U.S., good health is elusive and access to health care and prevention programs are often related to economic status, race or ethnicity, gender, education, disability, geographic location or sexual orientation.[2] Some examples of health disparities in minorities cited by the CDC and the Indian Health Service (IHS) include the following:

African Americans[2]

- Cancer—In 2001, the age-adjusted death rate for cancer was 25.4% higher for African Americans than for white Americans.
- Diabetes—In 2001, the diabetes age-adjusted death rate for African Americans was more than twice that for white Americans.
- Adult Immunization—In 2002, influenza vaccination coverage among adults 65 years of age and older was 70.2% for whites and 52 % for African Americans.

American Indians and Alaska Natives[3]

- American Indians and Alaska Natives die at higher rates than other Americans from alcoholism (770%), tuberculosis (750%), diabetes (420%), accidents (280%), suicide (190%), and homicide (210%).
- The American Indian and Alaska Native people have long experienced lower health status when compared with other Americans. Lower life expectancy and the disproportionate disease burden exist perhaps because of inadequate education, disproportionate poverty, discrimination in the delivery of health services, and cultural differences. These are broad quality of life issues rooted in economic adversity and poor social conditions.
- Chronic diseases—Heart disease and cancer are the leading causes of death among American Indians and Alaska Natives. The prevalence of diabetes is more than twice that for all adults in the U.S., and the mortality rate from chronic liver disease is more than twice as high according to 2002 data.[2]

Asian Americans[2]

- Asian Americans are people having origins in any of the original peoples of the Far East, Southeast Asia, or the Indian subcontinent. Asian American populations are generally concentrated in the western states, the Northeast, and part of the South.[4]
- Access to health care—According to the 2000 U.S. census, Asian Americans represent 4.2% of the U.S. population. Overall, about 21% of Asian Americans lack health insurance compared to about 16% of the general population.
- Asian Americans suffer disproportionately from certain types of cancer, tuberculosis, and Hepatitis B. The leading causes of death in the U.S. in 2001 for Asian Americans or Pacific Islanders were cancer, heart disease, stroke, unintentional injuries, diabetes, and chronic lower respiratory disease.[5]
- Asian Americans have the highest rates of liver and stomach cancer for men and women and the third highest incidence rates of breast, lung, colon and rectal cancer for women.[5]

Native Hawaiians and Other Pacific Islanders[2]

- Native Hawaiians are 2.5 times more likely to be diagnosed with diabetes than non-Hispanic white residents of Hawaii of similar age.
- Native Hawaiians in Hawaii have almost twice the rate of asthma compared to other races in the state.
- In 2000, infant mortality among Native Hawaiians was 9.1 per 1,000, almost 60% higher than among whites.
- Asian Americans and Pacific islanders had the highest tuberculosis cases rates of any racial and ethnic population in 2001.

Hispanic/Latino Americans[2]

- Hispanic or Latino is a person of Spanish, Mexican, Puerto Rican, Cuban, Central or South American or other Spanish culture. Hispanics are white, black, indigenous, Asian and every possible combination thereof, and originate from more than 20 countries. Hispanics are identified separately as an ethnicity; they can be of any race.
- Hispanics generally have lower mortality rates but higher morbidity rates compared with the overall U.S. population. As a result, morbidity and chronic disease management are areas of great concern for health care providers working with this population.[6]
- There are differences in morbidity rates for chronic diseases within or among the Hispanic population as well. Among Hispanics, the diabetes death rate in 2000 was highest among Puerto Ricans, followed by rates for Mexican Americans and Cuban Americans.
- Work related injuries—Mexican foreign-born workers accounted for 69% of the 2,440 fatally injured, foreign-born workers between 1995 and 2000.
- In 2002, influenza vaccination coverage among adults 65 years of age and older was 70.2% for whites and 46.7% for Hispanics.

Students should understand that when the pharmacist provider is perceived to be disinterested or less engaged in the patient-provider relationship, the patient is more likely to convey mistrust in you as the provider—not ask or respond to pertinent questions related to their care, refuse to accept treatment advice, and comply poorly with prescribed treatment. The pharmacist preceptor should educate students and make them aware that despite our best intentions, racial and ethnic disparities do exist in health care.

"The lack of minority health professionals is compounding the nation's persistent racial and ethnic health disparities. From cancer, heart disease, and HIV/AIDS to diabetes and mental health, African Americans, Hispanic Americans, and American Indians tend to receive less and lower quality health care than whites, resulting in higher mortality rates. The consequences of health disparities are grave and will only be remedied through sustained efforts and a national commitment."[7]

It is the intent of the authors in the sections to follow to provide some basic information relating to social and economics issues relating to health care, access to care, health literacy, and cultural competency for preceptors in order to enhance the students' understanding, knowledge, and skills in how cultural and social factors influence health care. By becoming aware of causal factors that could be eliminated or modified and application of appropriate knowledge and skills, we can improve the health status of all our patients.

References

1. Smedley BD, Stith AY, Nelson AR, eds. *Unequal Treatment: Confronting Racial and Ethnic Disparities in Health Care.* Institute of Medicine (IOM). Washington DC: National Academy Press; 2003.
2. Centers for Disease Control and Prevention (CDC). *Fact Sheet: Racial and Ethnic Disparities.* April 2004.
3. Indian Health Service. *Facts on Indian Health Disparities.* Cited September 2002.
4. Census Bureau. *Census 2000 Brief: Overview of Race and Hispanic Origin.* 2000.
5. Unites States Commission on Civil Rights. *The Health Care Challenge: Acknowledging Disparity, Confronting Discrimination, and Ensuring Equality.* September 1999.
6. Kaiser Permanente. *A Provider's Handbook on Culturally Competent Care: Latino Population.* Oakland, CA: Kaiser Permanente National Diversity Council; 2001.
7. The Sullivan Commission. *Missing Persons: Minorities in the Health Professions—A Report of the Sullivan Commission on Diversity in the Healthcare Workforce.* September 2004. Available at: http://www.sullivancommission.org. Accessed October 8, 2004.

Every man must decide whether he will walk in the light of creative altruism or the darkness of destructive selfishness. This is the judgment. Life's most persistent and urgent question is what are you doing for others?

Martin Luther King, Jr.

Understanding Social and Economic Issues Relating to Health Care

Nicanora C. Cuéllar

Objectives

- Identify legislative changes that have increased or decreased access to health care.
- Recognize recent economic trends that have reduced access to health care.
- Distinguish employer benefit decisions that are increasing consumer health care expenses.
- Understand that some populations are more vulnerable to having inadequate access to health services.
- Recognize that not having health care insurance can be financially devastating for individuals of all income levels.
- Support consumer health care and community resources self-management.
- Optimize financially-indigent and medically-indigent consumer use of available resources for free or discounted health services.

Social and Economic Aspects of Access to Health Care

The changing and difficult economic situation in the United States has resulted in a growing health care crisis affecting all socioeconomic and cultural groups. Providers can develop a more astute and compassionate health care practice if they endeavor to understand the increasing, similar and different social and financial challenges encountered by U.S. residents needing and seeking health care. The federal and state governments have addressed these issues through legislative changes promoting increased access to health care. However, these legislative changes have not sufficiently addressed the health care needs of the working poor and some middle-income workers. A growing number of workers are simultaneously struggling to meet daily living expenses and at the same time are overwhelmed with the financial burdens of paying for health insurance and/or chronic health care expenses. Health care providers can familiarize themselves with applicable laws and public benefits, cultural issues, intervention strategies, as well as available resources to decrease health care risk and promote more positive health care outcomes for their patients.

For many years the mounting health care crisis has been the focus of the U.S. federal government and a great concern to the American business community and workers. During the 1990s, the U.S. government under the Clinton Administration organized a national committee to develop a universal health insurance plan. This committee's proposals were not well-received by the insurance industry or by the medical community and failed to be voted into federal legislation. An important concern was whether the government, health care providers, or the individual patients themselves would be making health care decisions under the proposed universal health care plan.

Later in the 1990s, the Personal Responsibility and Work Opportunity Reconciliation Act (PRWORA) of 1996 altered eligibility criteria for public (federal welfare) assistance programs. The law's primary intent was to limit cash assistance to, and dependency by, needy families by promoting job preparation and work and by supporting the formation and preservation of two-parent families. Additionally, with the PRWORA uninsured nonqualified aliens (nonimmigrant visitors and undocumented immigrants) are limited to emergency Medicaid benefits and are left without health plan coverage for post-hospital discharge care (i.e., outpatient medical care, home health, inpatient rehabilitation, medical equipment and supplies, outpatient medications, and nursing home placement). Legal immigrants are currently ineligible for nonemergency Medicaid benefits for their first five years in the U.S. with some exceptions.*

The Balanced Budget Act of 1997 created the State Children's Health Insur-

---

*Exceptions: (1) refuges; (2) persons granted asylum and persons whose deportation is being withheld; (3) armed forces personnel or veterans and their dependent family members; (4) legal permanent residents with 40 Social Security qualifying quarters of work; and (5) those receiving Supplemental Security Income (SSI) benefits on August 22, 1996 and, subsequently, certified eligible under SSI as blind or disabled.

ance Plan (SCHIP). Under SCHIP each state offers health insurance for little or no cost for uninsured children up to the age 19 years. State regulations for income eligibility and health services vary under each state-administered CHIP. SCHIP was intended to bridge the gap for children living in households income-ineligible for Medicaid benefits but who nonetheless reside in households with gross family incomes at or below twice the federal poverty level.[†] Some states have enacted state legislation that provides more generous means tests. The recent downturn in the national economy since the beginning of the 21st century resulted in a reduction in federal and state funding, stalling congressional efforts to allow parents of SCHIP children to also be enrolled under SCHIP.

During the latter part of the 1990s, health uninsurance was reduced for low income and some low moderate-income children with the expansion of the Medicaid Program and the initiation of health care benefits for children under the federally mandated SCHIP. In a few states, parents of low-income children were allowed to enroll in federal health programs. Subsequently, federal and state budget shortfalls in the past several years resulted in federal and state program cutbacks affecting eligibility for low-income adults and children and compounding the health care crisis in the United States.[1] While children's uninsurance rates remained steady the past several years, cutbacks in organized outreach efforts and more complex application processes have likely resulted in eligible children not becoming enrolled or losing eligibility.[2]

Beginning in 2004, The Medicare Prescription Drug, Improvement and Modernization Act (DIMA) of 2003 provides drug discount cards for Medicare recipients and an additional $600 credit for those with low annual incomes. On January 1, 2006 Medicare drug discount cards will begin to be replaced by new Medicare prescription plans. Patients and their families can be directed to www.Medicare.gov for information on public and private programs that offer discounted or free medication, information on using generic medications and other means to reduce health care costs, and Medicare health plans that have prescription benefits.

The Family Medical Leave Act (FMLA) of 1993 provides workers of em-

---

[†]$37,700 is twice the federal poverty level for a family of four in 2004.

ployers with 50 or more employees up to a total of 12 (nonconsecutive) work-weeks of unpaid leave during any rolling 12-month period for the following: (1) the birth and care of a newborn child; (2) the new adoption of a child by the employee; (3) the care of an immediate family member (spouse, child or parent) with a serious health condition; or (4) medical leave when the employee is unable to work because of a serious health condition. For serious medical conditions, the employee using FMLA may be required to obtain medical forms from the ill family member's physician annually or as frequently as monthly. Some employers have bureaucratic procedures that make access to FMLA benefits difficult to obtain. Employees with available paid leave may be able to use vacation time and/or sick time to care for themselves or their family member. However, serious health conditions frequently result in employees taking unpaid medical leave, compromising already strained family finances.

In the U.S. there are more than 9 million parents who are uninsured. Working adults with gross family incomes at or below twice the federal poverty level represent two in five uninsured Americans. Employers are progressively shifting health care expenses to their employees. In the economic downturn of recent years, employers have increasingly decided to stop offering health care benefits to their employees or are offering plans that are less generous and inclusive. Most uninsured low-income adults either work at jobs that offer no health plan or cannot afford to participate in the high-cost health plan offered.[3]

Between the years 2000–2003, the number of uninsured adults grew by an additional 5 million. This has been as a consequence of a reduction in employer-sponsored insurance plans and the economic downturn that resulted in movement of workers from large firms to medium- or small-sized firms and to self-employment, which is less likely to offer health plans. Workers moving from full-time to part-time employment and from two-working parents to one-working parent households have also contributed to the growing number of uninsured adults. Increased uninsurance has affected low-, moderate- and high-income workers but mostly low-income young workers. Due to the recent economic recession, the ranks of low-income adults have increased with the shift of some middle-income adults to low-income status. It is anticipated that the rate of uninsured individuals will continue to increase with the trend of declining employer-sponsored health coverage.[1] Also, employers who maintain health coverage for their employees are incrementally increasing employee cost-sharing (i.e., increasing premiums, copays, coinsurance and costs of spousal and family coverage; thinning benefits, etc.).[4]

Racial and ethnic minorities in the U.S. have incomes and rates of health insurance coverage that are unequally lower compared with their white counterparts. Low income Hispanics, although more likely to have a stable (full-time) income across several years compared to other low-income groups, have the highest uninsured rates.[1] Thirty-seven percent of nonelderly Latinos are uninsured (87% of the uninsured Latinos are in working families) compared to 14% for whites. Sixty percent of Latinos reside in households below twice the federal poverty level compared to 23% of whites.[5]

Public policy (lack of increased funding for several years for the Indian Health Service [IHS]) has contributed to poor health, shorter life expectancies, and the frequency of disease for American Indians and Alaska Natives. Many Medicaid-eligible, low-income American Indians are not enrolled in Medicaid.[6] Eighty percent of American Indians do not have access to the IHS due to their residence in urban areas (have to travel to home reservation to receive IHS care) or because they belong to a nonfederally recognized tribe and nearly half have incomes below twice the federal poverty level.[7]

Eight in 10 African Americans reside in working families, but 23% are uninsured, 21% receive Medicaid benefits, and about half have family incomes below twice the federal poverty level. Their uninsured rates are about one and one-half times that of whites. The welfare reform of the 1990s transitioned many individuals into low-paying jobs with no or unaffordable health benefits. Transitional Medicaid benefits have been denied to families moving from public welfare programs to the workforce due to inadequate program administration and outreach efforts.[8]

Asian Americans and Pacific Islanders represent a number of widely diverse subgroups. For example, Korean Americans have 48% job-based health coverage while Japanese Americans have 77% coverage. These subgroups have different rates of self-employment and of work in small businesses (which are less likely to offer health benefits and are an important factor in uninsurance rates), citizenship, refugee status, income status, and participation in Medicaid despite rates of poverty that are higher than for the white U.S. population.[9]

Part-time employment and breaks in employment leave low-income families without coverage or with gaps in health care coverage. The Consolidated Omnibus Budget Reconciliation Act (COBRA) of 1986 allows some employees and their families who lose their health plan benefits due to specified circumstances (e.g.,voluntary or involuntary job loss, reduction in work hours, changes in jobs, death, divorce, and other life events) the right to continue group health coverage under the former employer's group health plan for limited periods of time. The cost is 102% of the entire premium (total of employer and employee expenses) and applies to group health plans sponsored by employers with 20 or more employees. However, the cost of COBRA benefits is cost-prohibitive for low- and moderate-income families already struggling to pay for basic family necessities due to job loss, underemployment, or part-time employment.

The Commonwealth Fund Biennial Health Insurance Survey revealed that gaps in health insurance coverage and large medical bills reduced individuals' ability to access appropriate health care.[1] About 20 million American families experienced problems in 2003 with paying medical bills; about one-third of these families were uninsured, and about two-thirds had health insurance. The presence of health coverage does not protect people from high out-of-pocket medical costs, and nearly half of all personal bankruptcies are due in part to medical expenses. Additionally, due to the economic recession of recent years, some state Medicaid programs have reduced benefits, imposed limits (i.e., monthly prescription limits), or imposed copays. About one-half of all families with medical bill problems are low-income. Almost two-thirds of all families with medical bill problems also reported difficulty with paying for basic family necessities (shelter, food, or transportation) due to medical debts.[10]

In 2003, 12.3 million working-age people (3 million uninsured) with chronic health conditions resided in families having problems in paying medical bills, making them more likely to delay or skip necessary medical care. Chronic conditions usually necessitate regular medical follow-up and higher out-of-pocket medical costs. Of the 3 million uninsured, 42% went without necessary care, 65% delayed care, and 71% went without needed prescriptions. Of the 12.3 million working-age people, 64% were contacted by a collection agency and 50% had to borrow funds. Recent studies have discovered that doubling of a copay from $10 to $20 resulted in significant cutbacks in the use of important prescription medications (i.e., diabetes and high cholesterol).[11]

Individuals with chronic health problems are frequently dependent on others for basic needs such as psychological support and medical transportation, and in more complex medical situations, for help with activities of daily living (bathing, dressing, mobility, and/or feeding). The frequency of medical appointments for the chronically ill person can result in lost income for the family member who must give up work hours or employment to care or provide support for the ill individual. When the adult providing support is the single or primary wage earner in the household, the combination of lost income and emotional stress of caring for the chronically ill person compounds family psychosocial stressors. If the adult providing support works for a small employer, there is an increased risk for job loss due to the employer being unable to accommodate the employee's work tardiness or absences.

It is important to consider that despite the differences between ethnic, age, and cultural groups noted above, people have many things in common. Also, an advantage of diversity and differences between individuals is that we can learn from our patients. Health care providers can improve access to health care and reduce health risk for their patients with even small but important endeavors such as providing warm, friendly greetings, as well as visual observation and active listening to perceive commonalities and health concerns. Health literacy assessments help providers understand how individuals learn about and adapt to their health problems and treatment plan. Consumer confidence and trust are promoted by the presentation of treatment issues in a manner that develops common health care goals. It is important to identify what patients hope to accomplish by jointly planning for treatment. Helping patients to understand and prioritize their treatment plan and health care strategies and to comprehend how health care outcomes will be measured is integral to collaborative patient-provider health care.

A strategy for improving the delivery of health care services is for preceptors and students to gain knowledge about the health care beliefs, values, and cultural communication etiquette of different ethnic groups (Table 8.1). Another essential approach is to take time to appreciate the individual's identity, literacy level, and degree of acculturation/assimilation (Table 8.2). The student's

Table 8.1 • *Objective: To gain knowledge about health care beliefs, values, and cultural communication customs of different ethnic groups.*

Strategies:

1. *Learn about attitudes regarding frankness about health problems (e.g., is it acceptable to speak to the patient or their family about prognosis, death and dying?)*
2. *Culturally, who is the decision-maker or head of the household?*
3. *Does the patient or family adhere to traditional non-American cultural practices or the American model (the patient or legal representative is responsible for health care decisions) of decision-making in health care?*
4. *Are there any characteristic or culture-specific meanings to particular health conditions and diseases?*
5. *Are there cultural norms regarding social distance, eye contact, communication, and physical contact between the genders or between the patient and health care provider?*
6. *Are health care decisions individual-centered or family-centered?*

Table 8.2 • *Objective: To appreciate the individual's identity, literacy level, and degree of acculturation/assimilation.*

Strategies:

1. *Evaluate own assumptions about who is a "good patient."*
2. *Assume mutual respect.*
3. *Greet patients and their families with a warm smile and steady handshake (when culturally appropriate).*
4. *Make physical contact (e.g., handshake, hand on the shoulder of an elderly person, pat on the head of a small child, etc.) with the very young, elderly, or infirm family members.*
5. *Ask where the patient and their family were born and how long they have been in the United States.*
6. *Inquire which languages they speak and are most comfortable talking and receiving written information in.*
7. *Ask the patient and/or family what concerns them most about the illness/disease.*
8. *Observe the patient or parent's ability to complete consent and intake forms to screen for potential learning and literacy issues.*

ability to assess the patient and family's abilities to comprehend and adapt to their disease management process is integral to understanding health literacy, health education, and compliance issues (Table 8.3). Finally, ascertaining and expanding the patient and family's knowledge and use of available resources provides the patient with an integral support system for successful self-management of his/her disease or acute or chronic condition (Table 8.4).

Table 8.3 • *Objective: Assessment of the patient and family's abilities to comprehend and adapt to their disease (integral to understanding health literacy, health education and compliance issues).*
Strategies:
1. Promote patient confidence.
2. Understand that an authoritarian posture decreases patient empowerment and participation and may increase dependency on the provider.
3. Ask about the patient's support system (e.g., who is available to provide financial support, emotional support, medical transportation, physical care, care of other family members, etc.).
4. Use social persuasion (family support).
5. Acknowledge that the patient or family may already be involved in health care self-management.
6. Reinterpret symptoms and recommendations as necessary.
7. Provide regular (re) assessment of progress and issues as well as goal-setting and problem-solving support.
8. Support the patient or family with setting specific, attainable health care goals.
9. Negotiate during health care encounters.

Table 8.4 • *Objective: Ascertain and expand the patient and family's knowledge and use of available resources to provide the patient with an integral support system for successful self-management and self-efficacy.*

Strategies:

1. *View patient encounters as opportunities for information-sharing and as a partnership with the patients and their families.*
2. *Assist with weighing the costs and advantages of the treatment options.*
3. *Language barriers are sometimes misinterpreted as noncompliance; therefore, obtain competent, nonbiased interpretive services to increase patient participation and satisfaction, as well as confidence, compliance, and positive outcomes.*
4. *Medicaid and CHIP are governmental programs that assist poor and low-income children and/or adults with health care expenses, which are accessed through state agencies.*
5. *Medicaid managed care health plan member services departments assist with providing on-site interpretive services.*
6. *Medicaid benefits include medical transportation services to medical appointments and to pick up prescription medications.*
7. *Drug company patient assistance internet sites include: www.rxassist.org; www.rxhope.com; www.needymeds.com; www.rxoutreach.com; www.helpingpatients.org; www.Medicare.gov/prescriptions/home.asp; www.TogetherRxAccess.com; and www.ashp.org/PAP/.*
8. *www.Medicare.gov assists with Medicare information on public and private programs that offer discounted or free medication, information on using generic medications and other means to reduce health care costs, and Medicare health plans that have prescription benefits.*
9. *Workers can obtain employer-specific or Department of Labor forms to request Family Medical Leave Act (FMLA) benefits from their human resources office.*
10. *Workers may be eligible for short-term and/or long-term disability and/or COBRA benefits through their employer's human resources office.*
11. *Individuals with terminal illness or severe disability expected to last 12 months or more may be eligible for Social Security Disability Income (SSDI) (may eventually receive Medicare benefits with this) or Supplemental Security Income (SSI) and Medicaid benefits from the Social Security Administration (1-800-772-1213 or www.ssa.gov/disability/).*

(continued)

Table 8.4 • *Objective: Ascertain and expand the patient and family's knowledge and use of available resources to provide the patient with an integral support system for successful self-management and self-efficacy. (continued)*

12. *Consumers with outstanding hospital bills may be eligible for hospital charity care or indigent care programs.*
13. *Consumer Credit Counseling Services (1-800-493-2222 or 1-800-388-2227, or www.moneymanagement.org) is an agency that helps consumers negotiate reasonable payment arrangements.*
14. *The state insurance commissioner's office may be able to provide information about high-risk insurance pools.*
15. *Local or state-wide hospital districts may be able to provide free or discounted health care services.*
16. *The Special Supplemental Nutrition Program for Women, Infants, and Children (known more commonly as the WIC Program) provides services to low-income infants, children up to the age of five years, and pregnant women. WIC services include nutritional supplements and free or very low-cost immunizations.*
17. *City and county health departments/clinics provide free or very low-cost immunizations and other health care services.*

References

1. Doty MM, Holmgren AL. *Unequal Access: Insurance Instability Among Low-Income Workers and Minorities.* The Commonwealth Fund. April 2004.
2. Holahan J, Ghosh A. *The Economic Downturn and Changes in Health Insurance Coverage.* Kaiser Commission on Medicaid and the Uninsured: The Urban Institute; 2000–2003.
3. Rosenbaum S, Sonosky C. *Policy Brief: Options for Assisting Uninsured Parents in Securing Basic Health Services.* The Commonwealth Fund. February 2002.
4. Regooulos L, Trude S. *Issue Brief. Findings from HSC. Employers Shift Rising Health Care Costs to Workers: No Long-Term Solution in Sight.* Center for Studying Health System Change. May 2004.
5. The Kaiser Family Foundation. *Kaiser Commission on Medicaid and the Uninsured Key Facts: Health Insurance Coverage and Access to Care Among Latinos.* June 2000.
6. Grantmakers Health. *Strategies for Reducing Racial and Ethnic Disparities in Health.* Issue Brief No. 5.
7. The Kaiser Family Foundation. *Kaiser Commission on Medicaid and the Uninsured Key Facts: Health Insurance Coverage and Access to Care Among American Indians and Alaska Natives.* June 2000.
8. The Kaiser Family Foundation. *Kaiser Commission on Medicaid and the Uninsured Key Facts: Health Insurance Coverage and Access to Care Among African Americans.* June 2000.

9. The Kaiser Family Foundation. *Kaiser Commission on Medicaid and the Uninsured Key Facts: Health Insurance Coverage and Access to Care Among Asian Americans and Pacific Islanders.* June 2000.
10. Mary JH, Cunningham PJ. *Issue Brief. Findings from HSC. Tough Trade-Offs: Medical Bills, Family Finances and Access to Care.* Center for Studying Health System Change. June 2004.
11. Tu HT. *Issue Brief. Findings from HSC. Rising Health Costs, Medical Debt and Chronic Conditions.* Center for Studying Health System Change. September 2004.

What you do speaks so loud that I cannot hear what you say.

Ralph Waldo Emerson

Enhancing the Student's Understanding of Health Literacy

Lourdes M. Cuéllar

Objectives

- Define health literacy.
- Describe the impact of poor health literacy on patients' health status.
- Demonstrate tools that preceptors and students can use to identify patients with low health literacy skills.
- Identify skills and tools that can be utilized to address problems with health literacy.

What is health literacy? *Healthy People 2010* defines health literacy as the degree to which individuals have the capacity to obtain, process, and understand basic health information and services needed to make appropriate health decisions.[1] More simply stated, it is the patient's ability to read, understand, and act on health care information. People with low health literacy are less likely to understand written and verbal information or instructions given to them by physicians, pharmacists, nurses, or insurance companies. They are frequently unable to follow directions such as those found on medication labels or appointment schedules.[1] Persons with the most health problems and the greatest need for self-management skills often have the poorest health literacy skills.[1]

Health care systems as we know them today have created an incredible challenge for persons with low health literacy skills. Health care providers and others rely heavily on the use of the written word to communicate. Directions on consent forms, instructions for surgery or procedures and medication directions can be complex making it difficult for persons with low health literacy skills. There is only one medication frequency instruction, "take one tablet daily," that is understood greater than 90% of the time. The direction "take one tablet twice a day" is understood less frequently. HIV positive adults with low functional health literacy miss more treatment doses than patients with high health literacy because they do not understand instructions on how to take their medications.[2] Research has shown that literacy is a stronger predictor of health status than age, income, employment status, education level, or racial or ethnic makeup of the individual.

According to the National Adult Literacy Survey (NALS),[3] 75% of Americans who reported having a chronic illness (>six months) had limited literacy. The survey estimated that as many as 44 million people in the U.S. cannot read a prescription label, read a bus schedule, or interpret directions on a map. In addition, 53 million more are marginally literate. The average American reads between the 8th and 9th grade levels. The NALS survey also illustrated that adults with low literacy in America are comprised of 41% English-speaking whites, 22% English-speaking African Americans, 22% Spanish-speaking Americans, and 15% other. Practitioners who have worked with low-literacy patients for years are often surprised at the poor reading skills of some of their most poised and articulate patients.[4]

Inadequate health literacy increases with age. Patients with low literacy skills frequently utilize emergency rooms for primary care services or primary care facilities and community-based health centers. Because they are unlikely to obtain preventive health services, patients with low literacy make more unnecessary follow-up visits, are more likely to be hospitalized, and are more susceptible to medical errors.[5]

Patients with poor health literacy are more likely to have a chronic disease and less likely to understand their condition and obtain the health care they need. Only 50% of low literate patients know the symptoms of hypoglycemia or the definition of a normal blood sugar. Sixty percent of low literate patients do not know that exercise could lower their blood pressure.[6] Low literate patients with asthma are less likely to know how to use an inhaler. Low literate mothers are less likely to know how to read a thermometer.

Nonadherence to prescribed medication therapy is a common problem especially for patients with chronic diseases because patients with low health literacy skills often have limited knowledge of their medical condition. The complexity of dosage frequency or medication administration can lead to poor medication adherence.[6]

Because pharmacists are usually readily accessible to most patients or consumers, they may often be in a position to be the first health care provider to recognize that a patient is having health literacy problems. Some of the more important skills that preceptors should teach their students are methods to assess their patient's functional health literacy.[7] In addition, students should learn to be alert for "red flags" that can identify problems in this area. For example, a patient may say "I forgot my glasses. Can you read the directions on the label to me?" or "I'll read this when I get home." Patients may make excuses, clown around or use humor, become quiet or passive, or pretend they can read.

The use of "brown bag" or medication reviews with patients can be helpful ways to identify and address problems with health literacy. Teach students to ask open-ended questions to assess if a patient is able to name his/her medications or explain why and when medications should be taken. Use this discussion to identify areas of confusion and to answer patients' questions. Knowing how frequently patients are refilling their medication can also provide a clue about their medication adherence. Be alert to patients who have difficulty expressing medical concerns or has no questions. Do not ask, "Do you understand?" Create an environment where patients are not embarrassed to ask you questions or express their concerns. Patients should feel comfortable in indicating to you that they do not understand the information you may be trying to convey. Speak clearly and use plain language; avoid medical jargon to explain medical information.

The most successful interventions for promoting medication adherence include the use of both written and verbal communication. Often using visual tools or pictures helps the patients understand the action or behavior that is being recommended. Students should be taught to choose words that are at the 6th grade level and that show respect for a patient's culture. For example, if you are working with a patient to try and reduce fat intake, introduce the subject by saying "cutting back" rather than "eliminating" or "changing" from the use of lard to vegetable oil. Many patients do not understand what it means to take a medication on an empty stomach or twice or three times a day. The communication should emphasize the desired behavior rather than medical or medication facts. Using the "teach-back" or "show me" methods with all patients are still reliable methods to determine the extent of patients' understanding the instructions for taking their medication.[4]

Be a role model to your students and show them patient-centered communication skills. Teach them to engage in a conversation *with* patients; do not dictate to patients. Demonstrate to students how to encourage patients to ask questions. Speak slowly and start with the most important information or message first. Use repetition and demonstrate when follow-up phone calls may be helpful. Teach them, when appropriate, to give instructions not only to patients, but also to family members or other caregivers. Most importantly, teach students to listen actively to their patients, to learn about, and to address their patients' concerns.

Teach students to print out directions or label medications with the time indicated. That way patients have clear directions to follow. For example, for twice-a-day directions you may indicate to take at 9 a.m. and 5 p.m. or 8 a.m. and 6 p.m. Tailor the medication schedule to fit a patient's daily routine. The use of colors as codes or the use of pictures such as the sun and/or the moon can be used to indicate morning and night. Likewise, the use of charts, calendars, and picture books may also be helpful.

When preparing written materials to give to patients make sure that the documents are easy to read; write information at a 5th or 6th grade reading level. For most of the population anything above an 8th grade level, especially if dealing with medical information or terms, may be too difficult. Make the document or information look easy to read. Use bullet points and short sentences, and have lots of white space on the document or leaflet. Remember, for elderly patients you want to print or use a larger font for any written material that you give to them. Keep a patient's culture in mind when developing written information for patients. For example, in some cultures a patient many respond or adhere to prescribed therapy if you say something is "important" rather than "helpful." If the patient is having difficulty understanding written or verbal directions, a good approach may be to say "Many people have trouble reading and remembering these instructions. How can I help you?"

Students should learn to deliver short concise messages. Patients usually remember less than 50% of the information provided during each encounter. Teach students to use common everyday language when speaking to their patients. Some common examples:[4]

- For pain or pain killer instead of analgesic
- Make bones stronger instead of osteoporosis
- By mouth instead of oral
- Swelling instead of edema
- Sore or painful joints instead of osteoarthritis
- Treat cancer instead of chemotherapy
- High blood pressure instead of hypertension

Students should know when and how to use an interpreter. Many health care providers rely on family members and coworkers to serve as interpreters. Use a skilled interpreter, one who is competent to interpret and translate medically related issues.

Coworkers or staff may overestimate their own skills and abilities especially when a patient wishes to expand the discussion or requests additional information. Even patients who are bilingual may choose to communicate in their first language when the issues are emotional or involve their health. Remember to teach students how to look for nonverbal cues that a communication problem exists.

In summary, a person with good health literacy skills should be able to do the following:

- Understand diagnosis or condition.
- Understand medication instructions (e.g., take on an empty stomach, what twice a day means, etc.).
- Repeat back health care information and demonstrate the ability to utilize tools to manage chronic conditions such as a glucometer.
- Understand consent forms and accurately complete standard screening forms.
- Initiate questions with health providers.
- Understand how to effectively use insurance.

Both preceptors and students must demonstrate good communication skills including empathy, listening, and appreciative inquiry. The first impression you make on your patients can make a big difference. Demonstrate an attitude of helpfulness, caring, and respect, and put patients at ease so that they feel comfortable in asking questions.

References

1. *Healthy People 2010: Understanding and Improving Health*. U.S. Department of Health and Human Services, Office of Disease Prevention and Health Promotion; November 2000.
2. Kalichman, SC, Benotsch E, Suarez T, et al. Health literacy and health-related knowledge among persons living with HIV/AIDS. *Am J Prev Med*. 2000;18(4):325–31.
3. Kirsch J, et al. *Adult Literacy in America: A First Look at the Results of the National Adult Survey (NALS)*. Department of Education; 1993.
4. Parker R, Williams MV, Davis T. *Low Health Literacy—You Can't Tell by Looking*. American Medical Association Foundation; 1999.
5. Baker DW, Parker RM, Williams MV, et al. The health care experience of patients with low literacy. *Arch Fam Med*. 1996;5(6):329–34.
6. Williams MV, Baker DW, Parker RM, et al. Relationship of functional health literacy to patients' knowledge of their chronic disease: a study of patients with hypertension and diabetes. *Arch Intern Med*. 1998;158(2):166–72.
7. Youmans SL, Schillinger D. Functional health literacy and medication use: the pharmacist's role. *Ann Pharmacother*. 2003;37:1726–9.

You must be the change you wish to see in the world.

Mahatma Mohandas Ghandi

Teaching Students the Rationale for Providing Culturally Competent Care

Lourdes M. Cuéllar

Objectives

- Define culture and cultural competency.
- Explain the importance of providing culturally competent care.
- Understand the role of patients' health beliefs, health seeking behaviors and practices, and their impact in the delivery of optimal patient care.

"Culture is a pattern of learned beliefs, values, and behavior that are shared within a group; it includes language, styles of communication, practices, customs, and views on roles and relationships. We all belong to more than one culture, which may, for example, be social, professional, or religious; the concept goes beyond race, ethnic background, and country of origin. Culture shapes the way we approach our world and affects interactions between patients and clinicians."[1]

The National Center for Cultural Competence (NCCC) defines culture as an integrated pattern of human behavior which includes thoughts, communication, languages, beliefs, practices, customs, courtesies, rituals, manners of interacting, roles, relationships, and expected behaviors of a racial, ethnic, religious, social, or political group.[2] The NCCC states that there are numerous reasons to justify the need for cultural competence in health care at the patient-provider level.[3] These include but are not limited to the following:

- The perception of illness and disease and their causes varies by culture.
- Diverse belief systems exist related to health, healing, and wellness.
- Culture influences help seeking behaviors and attitudes toward health care providers.
- Individual preferences affect traditional and nontraditional approaches to health care.

- Patients must overcome personal experiences of biases within health care systems.
- Health providers from culturally and linguistically diverse groups are underrepresented in the current service delivery system.

The U.S. Department of Health and Human Services (HHS) Office of Minority Health defines cultural competency as the ability of the health care providers and organizations to understand, respect, and respond effectively to the cultural and linguistic needs brought by patients to the health care setting.

◆ **Preceptor Pearls**

- Ask patients what language they prefer when discussing their medical care and in what language they prefer to receive any written health care information.
- When first interacting with patients who were born in another country, it is best to use their last name when addressing them.
- Do not be insulted if a patient does not look at you directly in the eye or fails to ask questions. In many cultures it is not respectful to look at another person, especially someone in authority or highly respected like a health care provider.

Pharmacy students must learn how to communicate with and provide direct patient care services to patients of varying cultures and health care preferences. Students and preceptors should be able to demonstrate understanding and respect for patients with differing health beliefs and health seeking behaviors and practices, thereby demonstrating cultural proficiency. Preceptors and students must appreciate their patients' cultural beliefs; this is critical in the delivery of optimal care.

Asian Americans represent a wide variety of languages, dialects, and cultures. They are as different from one another as individuals from non-Asian cultures. According to the 2000 census, Asians and Pacific Islanders are comprised of the following: 25.4% Chinese, 19.3% are Filipino,

◆ **PRECEPTOR PEARLS**

Culturally Sensitive Patient Assessment Questions

- What do you think caused your illness or problem?
- What do you call your sickness or illness? How severe is it?
- What problems has your illness caused you?
- What kind of treatment do you think you should receive?

Adapted from Kleinman A. *Patients and Healers in the Context of Culture.* The American Medical Student Association. Berkeley: University of California Press; 1980. http://www.amsa.org/programs/gpit/cultural.cfm. Accessed October 1, 2004.

17.6% are Asian Indian, 11.7% are Vietnamese, 8.3% are Japanese, and 4.2% are Pacific Islanders.[4] More than half (54%) of the Asian and Pacific Islander population live in the West, 17% live in the South, 18% in the Northeast, and 11% in the Midwest. Nearly 40% of Asian Americans residing in the U.S. live in California. The greatest percentages of Asians are in Honolulu, San Francisco, San Jose, San Diego, Seattle, and Los Angeles. Language is the most prominent barrier for Asians and Pacific Islanders. According to the 2000 census, 66% of Asians and Pacific Islanders speak a language other than English at home. About 38% of Asian Americans do not speak English fluently.[4]

Although Cuban Americans are often classified as Hispanics or Latinos, their customs and traditions differ from Mexican American, Central American, or South American. "Latinos/Hispanics come from different nations and cultures. According to the 2000 census, Latinos are classified as follows: 58.5% Mexican American, 9.6% Puerto Rican, 4.8% Central American, 3.8% South American, 3.5% Cuban American, 19.8% are other Latino/Hispanic. The largest concentration is in four cities: New York, Los Angeles, Chicago, and San Antonio."[5] Data from the Kaiser study indicates that about 60% of Hispanic adults speak Spanish at home, 20% are bilingual, and 20% are English dominant.[5] Kaiser data also indicates that Hispanics are the most likely to be uninsured. This is because the jobs held by many Hispanics do not provide health benefits (e.g., migrant workers, day laborers, housekeepers, etc.).

The national standards for culturally and linguistically appropriate services (CLAS) in health care were set forth by the U.S. Department of Health and Human Services Office of Minority Health in order to provide guidelines on policies and practices aimed at developing culturally appropriate systems of care.[6] The scope of these standards, the teaching approaches, and the challenges to consider when implementing these standards are applicable to all health professionals.

◆ **Preceptor Pearls**

Performing a Cultural Assessment

- Identify or assess the patient's level of ethnic identity (e.g., first versus third generation).
- Language or communication barriers.
- Influence of religion, spiritual beliefs, or supernatural effects on the patient's health belief system.
- Concerns about racial or ethnic discrimination or bias.
- Educational and literacy, including health literacy levels.
- Current economic status.
- Cultural health beliefs and practices.
- Influence of family in compliance to prescribed treatment plan.
- Influence of family in the medical decision-making process.

Cultural competence has evolved from the making of assumptions about patients on the basis of their background to the implementation of the principles of patient-centered care, including exploration, empathy, and responsiveness to patients' needs values and preferences.[1] It is important not to stereotype patients broadly based on their ethnicity or culture. Unfortunately, this frequently happens when our care is based on textbook methods of addressing patients within the same cultural population such as Hispanics, Asians, or African Americans. There is no *one* way to treat any racial or ethnic group.

There are many aspects relating to cultural competence that preceptors need to teach their students. These include fundamental knowledge such as concepts of race, culture, ethnicity, family structure, gender roles, religion, death, differing communication styles, and principals of disease management as they relate to certain cultures. Preceptors can demonstrate and teach effective communication skills, relationship building, language proficiency or effective use of interpreters, ability to differentiate varying views of illness and healing, and how to recognize culture related problems. Preceptors can teach students how to integrate the patients' beliefs into the overall treatment strategy or plan. Lastly, complementary and alternative medicine (CAM) has growing social, economic, and clinical significance in the U.S. It is important for pharmacist preceptors and students to understand the implications of CAM for their patients: what it is, who uses it, and why.

> ◆ **PRECEPTOR PEARLS**
>
> Unless you are thoroughly effective and fluent in conversational and medical terminology of the target language, always use qualified medical interpreters. This is especially important to ensure information is conveyed in a neutral and confidential manner. Speak slowly, not loudly, and look at the patient, not at the interpreter. Avoid interruptions. Do not use friends, family, or children for medical interpretation. Provide instructions in an organized format (list) and have patients repeat their understanding of the message that was delivered. Return to an issue if you suspect it was not clear or may have been misunderstood.

The National Center for Complementary and Alternative Medicine (NCCAM) defines CAM as a broad range of healing philosophies (schools of thought), approaches, and therapies that mainstream Western (conventional) medicine does not commonly use, accept, study, understand, or make available.[7] A few of the many CAM practices include the use of acupuncture, herbs, homeopathy, therapeutic massage, and traditional oriental medicine to promote well-being or treat health conditions. Many CAM therapies are called holistic, which generally means they consider the whole person, including physical, mental, and spiritual aspects.[8]

Reaching cultural competence is a continuous process. The following example illustrates some of the challenges that pharmacists and students may encounter. An elderly Iranian woman has been admitted to your hospital. Neither the patient nor her family reads, speaks, or understands English. Her Muslin faith requires modesty, and she may not be the primary decision maker in her health care. Appropriate services for this patient may include the following: the use of interpreter staff; written information materials and consent forms that have been translated to Farsi; appropriate food choices; and clinical and support staff who understand how to interact appropriately with the patient and family.

> ◆ **PRECEPTOR PEARLS**
>
> Ask patients if they are taking any home remedies (herbs, teas, etc.) or if they have sought advice for their condition from others including family, friends, or alternative healers (e.g., abuela, sobrador, or curandero).

Using this example, how would you teach students to interact with this patient and/or her family?

A second example could be an elderly African American patient whose blood pressure has been difficult to control since the doctor changed his therapy to a new medication. Preceptors can teach students how to assess the patient through a thoughtful and respectful inquiry, which may discover that a distant relative had been involved with the Tuskegee Syphilis Study. For many African Americans, the Tuskegee study became a symbol of their mistreatment by the medical community. Patients such as the one mentioned above may not adhere to medical advice because they do not understand or do not trust their provider.

> ◆ **PRECEPTOR PEARLS**
>
> In Hispanic and African American families, family can play an important role in assuring adherence to prescribed medication therapy or disease management.

During Ramadan, adult Muslims are required to refrain from taking any food, beverages, or oral drugs between dawn and sunset. Because Ramadan can occur in any of the four seasons, the hours spent fasting can vary from 11 hours to 18 hours per day. The first meal is usually taken immediately after sunset and the second might be taken shortly before dawn. Many Muslim patients with chronic diseases insist on fasting even though they do not have to do so.[9] These patients may choose to change the time and dosing of their medications without seeking advice from their physician or pharmacist. Students should be able to inform their Muslim patients about when they should take their medication with regard to their altered food intake (before, with food, or after).

> ◆ **Preceptor Pearls**
> When talking to patients where English is not their primary language, speak clearly and slowly using a caring tone of voice. When possible, use pictures to help patients understand; repeat message if necessary to assure understanding.

One of the most important traits that a preceptor can model for students is respect and understanding of their patients. Simple gestures such as using an appropriate title (e.g., Mr., Mrs., Señor, Señora, etc.), asking permission before touching the patient to take a blood pressure, honoring elders, and demonstrating respect for patients' culture can go a long way in establishing a positive patient-provider relationship. Learn how to demonstrate respect in various cultural contexts.

> ◆ **Preceptor Pearls**
> How a patient expresses pain can vary significantly between cultures as well as between men and women. In some cultures stoicism is expected.

Educate students how to thoughtfully assess their patients' health beliefs, health-seeking behaviors, and general health knowledge. Coach them in the skill of gathering important patient information without being judgmental. Be quick to apologize, and accept responsibility for culture missteps (e.g., calling a woman by her husband's last name). It is common for a woman to change her last name after marriage in the U.S. This is not common practice

> ◆ **PRECEPTOR PEARLS**
> Assess a patient's understanding by asking open-ended questions. Do not say "Do you understand?" Be alert to nonverbal clues that may help assess a patient's understanding of the information provided.

outside the U.S.) Encourage students to read and learn more about the history and culture of the patients they are serving.

Preceptors can teach students the skills needed to be able to implement services that are accessible to and appropriate for diverse patient populations. Understanding the social and cultural background of the patients you serve and the environment that they live in is critical to providing quality patient care services. It is important to demonstrate to students how culturally competent clinical encounters result in more favorable outcomes, increase the satisfaction of the patient, and enhance the patient-provider experience. Being culturally competent will not only make you a more effective provider, but it will also make you a provider of choice.

References

1. Betancourt, JR. Cultural competence—marginal or mainstream movement? *N Engl J Med.* 2004:351(10)953–4.
2. National Center for Cultural Competence. *Conceptual Frameworks/Models, Guiding Values and Principles.* Available at: http://gucchd.georgetown,edu//ncc/. Accessed June 18, 2004.
3. Cohen E, Goode TD. *Rationale for Cultural Competence in Primary Health Care.* Policy Brief 1. Washington, DC: National Center for Cultural Competence; 1999.
4. Kaiser Permanente. *A Provider's Handbook on Culturally Competent Care: Asian and Pacific Islander Population.* 2nd ed. Oakland, CA; Kaiser Permanente National Diversity Council; 2001.
5. Kaiser Permanente. *A Provider's Handbook on Culturally Competent Care: Latino Population.* 2nd ed. Oakland, CA; Kaiser Permanente National Diversity Council; 2001.
6. Department of Health and Human Services, Office of Minority Health. *National Standards on Culturally and Linguistically Appropriate Services (CLAS) in Health Care. Final Report.* 2001.
7. Kaczmarczyk JM, Burke, A. *Complementary and Alternative Medicine Issues in Serving Diverse Populations.* Module 7 of Cultural Competence in the Clinical Care of Patients with Diabetes and Cardiovascular Disease. Washington, DC: Health Resources and Services Administration, Bureau of Primary Health Care, and Institute for Healthcare Improvement; 2003.
8. U.S. Department of Health and Human Services (US DHHS). (2003a). *Complementary and Alternative Medicine: Issues in Serving Diverse Populations.* Draft curriculum module 5 for Cultural Competence in the Clinical Care Model Project. Health Resources and Services Administration, Bureau of Primary Health Care; 2001.
9. Aadil N, Houti IE, Moussamih S. Drug intake during Ramadan. *BMJ.* 2004;329:778–82.

Additional Resources

Betancourt, JR. *The Impact of Race/Ethnicity, Culture, and Class on Clinical Decision-Making. Module 4 of Cultural Competence in the Clinical Care of Patients with Diabetes and Cardiovascular Disease (2002).* Washington, DC: Health Resources and Services Administration, Bureau of Primary Health Care, and Institute for Healthcare Improvement; 2003.

Ferguson JA, Weinberger GR, Westmoreland LA, et al. Racial disparity in cardiac decision making. *Arch Internal Med.* 1998;158(13):1450–3.

Flaskerud JH, Uman G. Directions for AIDS education for Hispanic women based on analyses of survey findings. *Public Health Rep.* 1993;108(3):298–304.

Frederick Schneiders Research. *Perceptions of How Race and Ethnic Background Affect Medical Care: Highlights from Focus Groups*. Menlo Park, CA: The Henry J. Kaiser Family Foundation; 1999.

Gordon AK. Deterrents to access and service for Blacks and Hispanics: the Medicare hospice benefit, healthcare utilization, and cultural barriers. *Hospice J.* 1995;10(2):65–83.

McKenzie K. Racism and health. *Br Med J.* 2003;326:65–6.

Morales LS, Cunningham WE, Brown JA, et al. Are Latinos less satisfied with communication by health care providers? *J Gen Intern Med.* 1999;14(7):409–17.

Peterson ED, Wright SM, Daley J, et al. Racial variation in cardiac procedure use and survival following acute myocardial infarction in the department of veterans affairs. *JAMA.* 1994;271(15):1175–80.

Tocher TM, Larson E. Quality of diabetes care for non-English speaking patients: a comparative study. *West J Med.* 1998;168:504–11.

Uba L. Cultural barriers to health care for Southeast Asian refugees. *Public Health Rep.*1992;107(5):544–8.

van Ryn M, Burke J. The effect of patient race and socio-economic status on physicians' perceptions of patients. *Soc Sci Med.* 2000;50:813–28.

Wagner TH, Guendelman S. Healthcare utilization among Hispanics: findings from the 1994 minority health survey. *Am J Manag C.* 2000;6:355–64.

It is not book-learning young men need, nor instruction about this or that, but a stiffening of the vertebrae which will cause them to be loyal to a trust, to act promptly, concentrate their energies; do the thing—"Carry a message to Garcia!"

***Elbert Hubbard, from* A Message to Garcia**

Chapter 9

Career Advising

Steven H. Dzierba, Darlene M. Mednick, Kevin Purcell

Chapter Outline

Planning is bringing the future into the present so that you can do something about it now.

Alan Lakein

The Role of the Preceptor in Career Planning

Steven H. Dzierba

Objectives

- Understand how to create professionals who anticipate, create, and embrace change.
- Provide insight on how to instill accountability into young practitioners.

Elbert Hubbard stated in his classic book *A Message to Garcia* that bosses are continually looking for that one person who will do the job[1]—someone who will complete the mission without asking silly questions or hastily delegating the task to another. A preceptor can influence the future career of a student in a variety of ways.

A savvy mentor offers opportunities for student growth. Residencies are one way to instill the value of experience in young practitioners. Students need to know the value of their experiences and as a result the potential opportunities for promotion. Employees must prosper where they are planted to keep open opportunities for promotion.

Emphasize the Need for Experience

Students lacking specific experiences are at a disadvantage during selection processes because candidate interviews rely on past performance being an indicator of future performance. Early experiences should include working in small teams. This model is relied on regardless of the type of pharmacy practice chosen.

Professional Organizations

Involvement in professional organizations is one way to gain experience. Working in local, state, and national organizations will help develop skills needed for future roles. Young practitioners are given opportunities to develop their own relationships and networks through such work. Students need exposure to as many of the potential opportunities that will be available to them in the future.[2]

Share Experiences

A mentor should share personal and professional experiences with students. Examples of success and opportunities for improvement offer unique value. Every preceptor has lived through situations that would be helpful if imparted to the students. Share what has worked and what has not. Engage students in asking why things did or did not work.

Constantly Ask for Feedback

Creating students who are open to coaching is every preceptor's goal. We want students to continually look for feedback after completing tasks, for example, someone who actively asks these questions once completing an activity:

1. What did I do well?
2. What can I do better?
3. What should I start doing?
4. What should I stop doing?
5. What should I change?

Students or employees with this mindset will improve their performance daily. Those improvements will result in solidifying their places with employers.

Start with the End in Mind

Preceptors can help students start their careers by asking them to visualize the end of their careers. Some mentors may ask students for their five- or ten-year plans. Other methods may have more impact, such as developing an Obituary, a Life Purpose Statement, and a Principles of Practice Statement. Fred Eckel, professor at the University of North Carolina, has assisted many health-system leaders in this process. None of these documents are prepared easily, and much soul searching is required. Students are asked to write their personal Obituary, then a Life Purpose Statement, and then their Principles of Practice. All should be completed with appropriate time for reflection and rewarded after completion of each step. Life and work plans that fit their meaning and mission of life are written. This develops in practitioners a sense of pride and satisfaction in their chosen profession of pharmacy. Students walk away with a career plan that they developed and believe in. They can then implement this plan throughout their lives. Decision-making becomes clearer when detailed plans are known.

References

1. Hubbard E. *A Message to Garcia*. Originally published East Aurora, NY: Roycrofters; 1899. Bedford, MA: Applewood Books; 1993.
2. Giorgianni SJ. *Full Preparation: The Pfizer Guide to Careers in Pharmacy.* New York, NY: Pfizer Pharmaceutical Group; 2001.

All our dreams can come true, if we have the courage to pursue them.

Walt Disney

Careers in Pharmacy

Darlene M. Mednick

Objective

- Identify and discuss the different careers opportunities available for pharmacists.

Many task forces and publications have cited the diversity of career opportunities for pharmacists as a reason for the workforce shortage that is occurring. More accurately, the more significant reasons are well-documented by various experts, including Dean David A. Knapp who authored the *Pharmacy Manpower Project*, and Dr. Katherine Knapp (no relation) who developed and has published widely on the Aggregate Demand Index. The drivers for this shortage have allowed organizations to better handle (or grapple) with the realities faced for what is reported to continue through 2020.

Regardless of the reasons for the pharmacist shortage, the diversity of career opportunities signifies a wonderful opportunity for pharmacists to choose thoughtfully between practice settings, taking into consideration their unique talents, interests, skills and competencies, along with balancing personal and professional life.

The variety of choices today versus the more historical and limited choices, has created greater challenges for practicing professionals (and employers of pharmacists) to create work environments that understand and reflect the educational achievements and growing generational diversity.

Pharmacists face many challenges today. The most significant are the aging population, the increasing use of medications, direct-to-consumer advertising, more patient care being delivered in an outpatient setting, and the need to truly manage the drug therapy and disease states of patients.

Many pharmacists have sought practice settings that more fully utilize their skills and allow for growth in their careers. All of these present pharmacists with many opportunities beyond the more traditional product-based dispensing, distribution, and delivery of medications. In fact many of these newer nontraditional practice settings have been an important driver for the changing roles we now see.

While it is true that the diversity of practice settings and career opportunities for pharmacists has never been greater, it is a remarkable advancement of the profession, which allows for highly talented and motivated pharmacists to exist at many important points along the health system continuum. Thus, it is even more important now that faculty, preceptors, mentors, and residency program directors be as familiar as possible with these opportunities in order to provide guidance to students and to allow for a match of skills/competencies and personal desires or objectives.

While it is somewhat human nature to excite someone about your own career path or choices and views, it is a real disservice to students or residents to overlook their unique characteristics and desires and instead create mirror images of ourselves.

The following information outlines current practice settings available to pharmacists, yet the opportunities will continue to expand given the ever-changing health care system in the U.S.

Many pharmacists traditionally begin their career in community- or hospital-based practice settings. Both settings have evolved to embrace the concept of pharmaceutical care where pharmacists are directly responsible for achieving definite outcomes that improve a patient's quality of life. In addition, the concept of pharmaceutical care has reached in both directions—backward and forward—to allow pharmacists to be involved in the development of clinical programs and decision-making for plan benefit programs administered by managed care organizations (MCOs), including PBMs (Pharmacy Benefit Managers).

Technology has also been an important part of health care leading to more career opportunities for pharmacists as seen in the increasing number of internet pharmacies and the growth of electronic prescribing and electronic medical/health record (EMR/EHR) companies. It becomes an even bigger factor as the Medicare Prescription Benefit is implemented.

The following are examples of careers/practice settings available to pharmacists:

- Community pharmacy
  - Compounding
- Institutional (hospital) pharmacy
  - Drug information
- Home care/LTC (long-term care) pharmacy
- Managed care pharmacy
- Pharmaceutical industry
  - Regulatory affairs
- Academia
- Research
- Consultant pharmacy
- Government
  - Civic and political leadership
  - Military
- Nuclear pharmacy
- Infectious diseases pharmacist
- Psychiatric pharmacy
- Nutrition
- Oncology
- OR pharmacist
- Pediatric pharmacist
- Poison control
- Veterinary pharmacist
- Professional associations
- Employee benefit consulting
- Clinical Research Organizations (CROs)
- Medical marketing and communication organizations
- Pharmaceutical and health care distributors
- Health care information technology companies

In almost all of these settings, pharmacists collaborate with physicians and other health care professionals to develop, implement, and monitor a therapeutic plan that ensures satisfactory clinical, economic, and humanistic outcomes.

Community Pharmacy

This is a familiar practice setting to everyone. It employs a large number of pharmacists—in fact 6 out of 10 pharmacists provide care to patients in a community setting.[1] Pharmacists in a community setting provide information and advice on health, provide medications and associated services, and refer patients to other sources of help and care when necessary. Many community pharmacies have developed specialties in DMR (durable medical equipment), homeopathic medicine, and compounding.

Community pharmacists also assist patients in understanding their prescription benefit program and provide disease and care management in a variety of areas, including diabetes, asthma, hypertension, and hyperlipidemia. Many pharmacists achieve specialty certifications in these key disease areas in order to better educate and assist patients in managing their health care.

Pharmacists with appropriate skills have also helped their organizations to design and implement technology solutions—robotics and other automation—to improve the quality, safety, and efficiency of the care they provide.

Unfortunately, many community pharmacy practice settings have continued to utilize pharmacists in a more traditional dispensing role rather than to fit these other activities into their operational and business model.

Management opportunities also exist—people, processes, and programs—for those with interest and skills/competencies. While many of these skills/competencies can be achieved through experience or on-the-job training, additional training in areas of business, process engineering, quality tools, and leadership is necessary in achieving these types of positions.

Institutional (Hospital) Pharmacy

There has been an increased need for pharmacists to provide care through organized health care settings, including hospitals, nursing homes, extended care facilities, neighborhood health centers, and ambulatory care clinics. While pharmacists work in these settings as drug information experts and systems control experts, they are also responsible for controlling drug distribution and systems to ensure that patients receive the appropriate medications. Many pharmacists continue to chair P&T committees as well as prepare drug monographs and therapeutic class reviews. Developing Drug Utilization Review (DUR) programs and performing DUR, as well as educating other health care professionals within the organization, are yet another large component of a hospital pharmacist's role and responsibilities.

The focus on medical errors brought to the forefront by the Institute of Medicine reports (*To Err Is Human: Building a Safer Health System* and the subsequent report *Crossing the Quality Chasm*) has enabled pharmacists who have a systems aptitude to become involved in organization- or enterprise-wide teams and address issues such as CPOE (Computerized Physician Order Entry) and quality checks within automated systems.

Pharmacists typically work with physicians and nurses in a collaborative team environment to provide direct patient care. These roles require pharmacists to possess additional competencies such as excellent communication skills, influence and persuasion, negotiation skills, and critical-thinking/problem-solving skills.

Many pharmacists in institutional practice as well as other practice settings specialize in the following areas, each requiring additional training (specialty residency and/or board certification):

- Nuclear pharmacy
- Infectious diseases
- Psychiatry
- Nutrition
- Oncology
- Internal medicine
- Cardiology
- Nephrology
- Geriatrics
- Critical care pharmacy
- Pediatrics
- Poison control
- Primary care

Long-Term Care Pharmacy

Pharmacists practicing in long-term care practice settings are responsible for drug information, education, and drug therapy management of a growing segment of our population. This area of pharmacy is practiced in home care agencies, adult day-care centers, hospices, and other long-term care facilities.

These patients often require DUR and adjustments to drug therapy due to diminished hepatic and renal functions, and to the fact that they are often the highest utilizers of drugs. With the increased use of medications and longer life expectancies, along with the Baby-Boomer population "wave" aging, specialization in geriatric pharmacy is expected to grow rapidly.

Managed Care Pharmacy

This area of pharmacy practice has grown dramatically over the last decade due to the need to manage the increase in health care expenditures, especially the double-digit trend in drug costs. Providing a prescription drug program as a part of the medical benefit has become increasingly difficult for many employers and other payers who recognize the importance of providing access to prescription drugs.

Many payers (government, employers, etc.) contract with MCOs (managed care organizations), including health plans and pharmacy benefit managers (PBMs), to help manage the quality, cost, and access of a prescription drug benefit. The primary goal is to ensure that what is spent on prescription drugs is appropriate and safe, as well as to ensure that medications are properly used. There are over 18,000 pharmacists practicing in a managed care setting.[2]

Managed care pharmacists are responsible for plan design; clinical program development; clinical management; pharmacoeconomics; outcomes research; communication and education of patients, prescribers, and pharmacists; and drug distribution and dispensing, as well as performing the clinical interventions to support the DUR, formulary management, and disease management of the populations that MCO serves. Pharmacists are also now more involved in the development, administration, and management of the pharmacy provider networks that provide care to patients, as well as in the performance and quality monitoring, reporting, auditing, and contracting of the network and services.

Another area within a health plan or PBM where a pharmacist's unique skills are valued is in the pharmaceutical contracting group. There, pharmacists monitor manufacturers' drug pipelines and develop forecasting models to determine the impact of that drug on a payer's program. In addition, they are often responsible for the clinical assessment and evaluation of the product, negotiation of the purchasing or utilization contracts, the programs designed to maximize the formulary, and recommendations for formulary decisions and administration.

Several large employers and insurers have also recognized the value and expertise of pharmacists in designing and managing a benefit and have hired pharmacists as a part of their managed medical team, many taking on roles of Chief Pharmacy Officer (CPO)—similar to the CMO (Chief Medical Officer)—within the management team. The integration of pharmacy into the medical strategy is very important in achieving the goals of quality, cost management, and access.

Many MCOs utilize mail order or online services as a management tool within the benefit. This creates opportunities for pharmacists as managers of operations (pharmacies owned and operated by the MCO or contracted entities), as well as specialists in key areas like targeted DUR programs, formulary management (including generic and therapeutic substitution), and disease management programs.

In addition, managed care pharmacists are involved with several patient safety programs including the following:

- DUR programs
- Prior authorization, developing step-therapy clinical rules or protocols
- Monitoring programs
- Quality assurance (QA) programs
- P&T committees
  - Pharmacoeconomics
  - Evidence-based medicine/clinical guidelines
- Communication/education programs
- Disease management/drug therapy management (DTM)
- Plan benefit design
- Compliance programs—addressing adherence and persistency with drug therapy

More detailed information is available at www.amcp.org/professional_res/concepts/index_concepts.asp.

Specialty Pharmacy

Managing biotechnology and self-administered injectables is a growing area of concern for many MCOs due to the complexity of the drug administration, need for specific patient education/management, and product storage. The cost of these drugs is usually very high and, therefore, ensuring proper use, administration, storage, and management is important.

Until recently these self-administered drugs have often been paid for as part of the medical benefit and have not been managed as unique products requiring additional services. There is a growing trend to "carve out" the management of these drug products usually through the PBM or health plan. As a result, there is an increasing number of specialty pharmacy organizations who focus only on the management of these drug therapies. The growth is directly related to the required, related services due to the complexity of therapy and the need for patient education, as well as to the growing number of biotechnology drugs available to treat diseases.

This provides pharmacists with another area of specialty practice focused on supporting patients living with complex health conditions. This includes education on the storage, administration, and special handling and delivery requirements for these expensive and difficult to find medications. Also, pharmacists are important in the clinical program development for these following products and interventions for complicated diseases:

- Acromegaly
- Chronic granulomatous disease
- Cystic fibrosis
- Gaucher disease
- Growth hormone disorders
- Viral hepatitis
- HIV/AIDS
- Infertility
- Multiple sclerosis
- Oncology-related conditions
- Psoriasis
- Rheumatoid arthritis
- Solid organ transplant

With the growing number of biotechnology products available and/or expected and the advent of pharmacogenomics, this is certainly an exciting time for pharmacists who want to utilize their clinical and business management skills.

Pharmaceutical Industry

The pharmaceutical industry represents many opportunities for pharmacists. It is not only broad in its offerings, but it is also continuing to evolve. Currently pharmacists hold positions in sales, training and education, clinical research and product development, marketing, outcomes research, pharmacoeconomics, regulatory affairs, epidemiology, clinical trials, and administration. Many pharmacists involved in pharmaceutical companies go on to obtain postgraduate degrees in order to meet the technical demands and scientific duties required in pharmaceutical manufacturing and general business management.[1]

Pharmacists with an interest in sales and administration can combine their clinical expertise in positions such as medical service representatives or liaisons, or clinical educators. Like many other organizations, specifically MCOs, the roles for pharmacists have grown tremendously, but industry pharmacists rarely have patient contact.

Great opportunities exist for pharmacists who have previously practiced in an MCO, due to their unique experiences and knowledge of managed care. They are increasingly valuable to the pharmaceutical industry as their customers/clients have shifted from physicians to MCOs. Many pharmaceutical companies have developed specific managed care divisions. These positions can lead to key positions for pharmacists who, understanding that market segment, can help them position and understand their product's placement on drug formularies, which incorporate many divisions from the brand team to pharmacoeconomics to medical information.

Another growth opportunity within the pharmaceutical industry is the medical information group, which is responsible for off-label drug information questions and the preparation of the product dossier that is a required part of the *Format for Formulary Submission*.[3] Similar opportunities exist in generic drug companies as well as in wholesale drug companies.

Academia and Research

Pharmacists who are full-time faculty members currently number approximately 3,000. These individuals are responsible for the teaching and education of the future members of the profession. Many faculty hold administrative and management positions within the university or college. They are also involved in research; public service; consulting to local, state, national and international organizations; and patient care.

Becoming a member of the faculty at a college of pharmacy usually requires a postgraduate degree and/or training (e.g., Ph.D. or residency or fellowship training following the professional degree program).[1]

In addition to teaching and research, pharmacy practice faculty have patient care responsibilities and are called educator/practitioners who precept students during internships and clerkships (experiential rotations). Other areas where pharmacists hold faculty positions are pharmaceutical sciences research (where an expertise in study design, methodology, and analytics is required to solve complex problems of drug utilization management) health care delivery, marketing, management, and other practice issues.[1] "Perhaps no other job in pharmacy has such far-reaching effects on the profession as that of an educator. It is in academia that one can excite individuals about pharmacy and lay the groundwork for continuing advances in the field."[1]

Consultant Pharmacy

Consultant pharmacists provide expert advice on the use of medications by individuals or within institutions, or on the provision of pharmacy services to institutions. The phrase "consultant pharmacist," coined by George F. Archambault who is referred to as the founding father of consultant pharmacy, originated in the nursing home environment when a group of innovative pharmacists focused on improving the use of medications in these facilities. However, consultant pharmacists are found today in a wide variety of other settings, including subacute care and assisted-living facilities, psychiatric hospitals, hospice programs, and in-home and community-based care.[4]

In addition to the more traditional definition and description above, there are increasing numbers of experienced pharmacists who consult in a variety of areas of expertise from managed care, to specialty disease areas or populations, to electronic prescribing and plan design.

Government

Traditionally pharmacists can be employed in staff and supervisory positions by the government at the Federal level, in the Departments of Public Health Service, the Veterans Administration, the Food and Drug Administration, and the Armed Services. At the state and local levels they are employed by regulatory, health, and social service agencies, including agencies charged with regulating the practice of pharmacy to preserve and protect the public health. As some state health agencies are consolidating their purchases, pharmacists are engaged in procuring supplies for the entire state. Some positions provide commissioned officer status others are under civil service. Many pharmacists hold positions within state Medicaid programs, especially in the DUR boards formed by many states.

Additional important and exciting opportunities are beginning to take shape due to the passage of the Medicare Prescription Drug, Improvement, and Modernization Act (MMA) of 2003. Already there are several pharmacists who have been hired at CMS (Centers for Medicare and Medicaid) and who have served as experts and committee leaders for NCVHS.

Professional Associations

Pharmacists also have careers in state and national professional associations. Several national professional associations are led and staffed by pharmacists with an interest and special talent in organizational work, including educational programming and services, meeting planning and management, writing, project management, research, and fundraising.

Below are some of the largest and most well-known associations:

- ASHP—American Society of Health-System Pharmacists
- APhA—American Pharmacists Association
- AMCP—Academy of Managed Care Pharmacy
- ASCP—American Society of Consultant Pharmacists
- ACCP—American College of Clinical Pharmacy

Employee Benefit Consulting

As mentioned in the managed care section, payers are facing a real challenge in providing a health care benefit, and there is an increased focus on the prescription drug program. Typically payers do not have the clinical expertise in-house and have been using benefit consultants (e.g., Mercer, AON, etc.) to help with plan design and benefit management, as well as their expertise and knowledge in selecting a PBM (Pharmacy Benefit Manager). Many even continue to use these organizations to manage the PBM relationship. Pharmacists with managed care and business experience are finding rewarding careers in these benefit consultant organizations as clinical program managers, account or client service managers, and as in-house expertise in developing and reviewing PBM services and contracts.

Contract Research Organizations (CROs)

Contract Research Organizations (CROs) design, manage, monitor, and analyze preclinical and clinical trials. These services are provided to the pharmaceutical industry and are increasingly valuable because the clinical trials are the basis for determining the safety and efficacy of pharmaceuticals, biologics, and medical devices. These organizations have gained popularity and growth over the last five years and have recently been attacked in the media due to the lack of expertise in-house. CROs will continue to provide career opportunities for pharmacists, especially in the Phase IV clinical trials required by the FDA.

Medical Marketing and Communication Organizations

Many pharmacists who excel at written and verbal communication skills have found exciting careers at medical communications companies, which develop clinical content for educational and promotional programs and publications for clinical and management professionals (e.g., Bimark Communications). Positions are staff and supervisory in the following areas: medical writing, program development, project management, clinical education, meeting planning and management, strategy, facilitation, business development, and account management.

Pharmaceutical and Health Care Distributors

Pharmacists in these organization ensure that the products needed to diagnose, prevent, and treat illnesses are distributed to the appropriate locations. In addition to the delivery of these products, many pharmaceutical and health care distributors have expanded their service offerings to include information, programs, and systems to make their customers more efficient and effective.

Pharmacists play a valuable role in all of these expanded services from designing and developing the programs, to the implementation and delivery of them and the systems necessary to manage them. Distributors are a vital force in saving consumers over $50 billion annually by reducing health care transactions and their associated costs.[5]

Pharmaceutical and health care distributors protect the quality and security of the products distributed. They also provide economies of scale to reduce distribution expenses, manage inventories to ensure product availability, and simplify distribution to ensure vital medication is available where and when it is needed.

Health Care Information Technology Companies

Many students and new practitioners are very familiar and comfortable with technology. In fact, many utilize online resources more frequently than any other resource, often citing the internet and company websites over more traditional sources of information. Therefore, it stands to reason that many are interested in careers that combine technical pharmacy knowledge with technology to deliver more integrated, efficient, and safe health care. In addition to health care information technology companies, a growing number of electronic prescribing companies, offering electronic medical records (EMRs) and electronic health records (EHRs), employ pharmacists as domain experts or in program development and management.

There are also organizations such as SureScript and RxHUB that are involved in developing electronic standards and the "highway" to address the fact that 44,000 to 98,000 Americans die each year as a result of medical errors. This statistic is associated with a cost of $17 to $29 billion and ranks medical error the eighth-leading cause of death in the United States. Medication errors in our nation's 7,000 hospitals can cost as much as $15 billion per year, accounting for over 770,000 injuries.

The goal of the health care industry is to enhance patient safety by accelerating the adoption of information technology. This is especially evident in the new MMA provisions on e-prescribing and in the President's mandate for electronic health records for all Americans by 2015. Pharmacists can play a significant role in helping to design, develop, and implement prescribing standards within information technology companies. They can also play an important role in bringing together health care providers and professionals in achieving this goal.

Dr. Barbara G. Wells, president of AACP and dean of The University of Mississippi School of Pharmacy, said "there's a crying need for pharmacists in all roles." She could not have said it better!

References

1. Purdue University, School of Pharmacy and Pharmaceutical Sciences. Becoming a pharmacist: career opportunities for pharmacy. Available at: www.pharmacy.purdue.edu/students/prospective/careeropts.php.
2. Academy of Managed Care Pharmacy. The role of pharmacists in managed health care organizations. Available at: www.amcp.org.
3. www.amcp.org or www.fmcp.org.
4. www.ascp.com. Accessed November, 9 2004.
5. www.aacp.org. Accessed November, 9 2004.

Additional Resources

Academy of Managed Care Pharmacy. The roles of pharmacists in managed health care organizations, Format for formulary submission, Framework for drug therapy management: a quality improvement tool, and Putting the pieces together: a pharmacy student's guide to managed care pharmacy. Available at: www.amcp.org. (800) TAP-AMCP.

American Association of Colleges of Pharmacy. Available at: www.aacp.org or www.pharmcas.org. (703) 739-2330. Accessed November 7, 2004.

American Association of Colleges of Pharmacy. Knapp DA. Professionally determined need for pharmaceutical services in 2020: a report of a consensus conference sponsored by Pharmacy Manpower Project, Inc. Available at: www.aacp.org. Accessed November 9, 2004.

American College of Clinical Pharmacy. Available at: www.accp.com. (816) 531-2177.

American Pharmacists Association. Available at: www.aphanet.org. (202) 628-4410.

American Society of Consultant Pharmacists. Available at: www.ascp.com. (703) 739-1300.

American Society of Health-System Pharmacists. Available at: www.ashp.org. (301) 657-3000.

Berlex. Inc. Berlex pharmacy careers. Available at: www.berlex.com/html/careers/pharma.

bhpr.hrsa.gov/healthworkforce/reports/pharmacist.htm.

National Association of Chain Drug Stores. Available at: www.nacds.org. (703) 549-3001.

National Community Pharmacists Association. Available at: www.ncpanet.org. (703) 683-8200.

National Pharmaceutical Association. Available at: www.npha.net. (800) 944-6742.

Pfizer, Inc. Pfizer's full preparation: the Pfizer guide to careers in pharmacy. Available at: www.pfizercareerguides.com.

The Pharmacist Workforce Shortage: A Study of the Supply and Demand for Pharmacists/ Dept HHS. http://bhpr.hrsa.gov/healthworkforce/reports/pharmacist.htm.

U.S. Department of Labor/Bureau of Labor Statistics/Bulleting 2540. Occupational outlook handbook, 2004–05 ed. Available at: www.bls.gov/oco/print/ocos079.htm.

www.aonconsulting.com.

www.bimarkcommunication.com.

www.mercer.com.

www.pharmacy.purdue.edu/students/prospectivecareeropts.php.

It is what you learn after you know it all that counts.

John Wooden

The Role of Pharmacy Residencies and Fellowships

Kevin Purcell

Objectives

- Identify ways for students to lead.
- Discuss mechanisms to develop lifelong learners.
- Define, contrast, and provide general information on residencies and fellowships.
- Provide a viewpoint on the increasingly important role of pharmacy residency and fellowship programs within the context of the changing U.S. health care system.

The health care environment has become more complex and the scope of pharmacy practice has broadened. Graduation from a Doctor of Pharmacy degree program provides pharmacists with minimum entry-level competency to practice pharmacy in a variety of settings. However, pharmacists who want to attain advanced clinical practice and pharmacy administration positions and best prepare themselves for future opportunities and leadership positions should consider completing a pharmacy residency. Increasingly, many employers (e.g., hospitals, clinics, managed care organizations) are seeking pharmacists who have completed an accredited residency. Pharmacists who wish to begin a successful research-oriented career should complete a pharmacy fellowship. Many universities and pharmaceutical companies are particularly interested in hiring pharmacists who have completed an accredited fellowship.

A pharmacy residency is an organized, directed, postgraduate training program in a defined area of pharmacy practice.[1] There are two major divisions of pharmacy residencies: (1) pharmacy practice residencies, and (2) specialized pharmacy residencies. The American Society of Health-System Pharmacists

(ASHP) is the primary organization responsible for residency program accreditation. ASHP also jointly accredits pharmacy practice residency programs with the American Pharmacists Association (APhA) and the Academy of Managed Care Pharmacy (AMCP). ASHP jointly accredits pharmacotherapy specialty residencies with the American College of Clinical Pharmacy (ACCP).[2]

Pharmacy practice residencies are sometimes referred to as the first year of postgraduate training (PGY1). They are one year in duration and can be completed in a variety of settings, including hospitals, health systems, managed care organizations, long-term care facilities, home health care organizations, and community pharmacies.[2] Their objective is to develop the resident's competence, skills, and application of drug therapy knowledge in providing the broad scope of pharmaceutical services needed in a practice setting.[2] The emphasis is on direct patient care and practice management, the progressive development of clinical judgment, decision-making skills, and leadership ability that began during the early and advanced experiential programs in pharmacy school.[2] Residents are held responsible and accountable for pursuing optimal medication therapy outcomes in patients under the supervision and guidance of role model practitioner preceptors.[2]

Pharmacy specialty residencies are sometimes referred to as the second year of postgraduate training (PGY2). They are usually one year in duration and are offered in a variety of specialty areas, including primary care, internal medicine, pediatrics, geriatrics, infectious diseases, critical care, oncology, psychiatry, pharmacotherapy, nutrition support, nuclear, drug information, and management.[2] Some residencies are two years in duration because they are combined with a master's degree (e.g., management) or they also encompass the requirements of the pharmacy practice residency (e.g., pharmacotherapy). Their objective is to develop the resident's competence, skills, and application of knowledge in a focused area of pharmacy practice.[2] Pharmacy specialty residencies build on the fundamental pharmacy practice responsibilities learned in a general pharmacy practice residency.[2] The emphasis is on developing expert knowledge and skills in a specialized area of pharmacy practice, far beyond what might be expected from a pharmacy practice residency.[2]

A pharmacy fellowship is a directed, highly individualized, postgraduate program designed to prepare the participant in becoming an independent researcher.[1]

Fellowships are usually two years in duration, based in pharmacy schools and academic health centers, and offered in a variety of specialty areas, including ambulatory care, clinical pharmacology, toxicology, neurology, nephrology, cardiology, drug development, pharmacogenomics, outcomes research, pharmacoeconomics, pharmacoepidemiology, pharmacokinetics, pediatrics, geriatrics, infectious diseases, critical care, oncology, psychiatry, pulmonary, transplantation, and women's health.[3] The emphasis is on developing the fellow's ability to conduct collaborative research and to function as a principal investigator.[3] Fellowships are about 80% devoted to research and typically include graduate coursework on research design and biostatistics.[3] Fellows are expected to already possess knowledge and practice skills relevant to the clinical area of the fellowship, which should have been obtained through practice experience or a pharmacy specialty residency.[3] The preceptor should be an established researcher.[3]

Information about residencies can be obtained on the ASHP website (www.ashp.org), including definitions, accreditation standards, a directory of accredited programs, the resident matching program, the residency showcase, links to the regional residency conference websites, and federal funding. Information about fellowships can be obtained on the ACCP website (www.accp.com), including definitions, guidelines and peer review for fellowships, and a listing of fellowships and residencies. Residency information and listings of managed care pharmacy residencies and community pharmacy residencies are available on the AMCP website (www.amcp.org) and the APhA website (www.aphanet.org), respectively. Additional information about residency programs can be obtained by attending the ASHP National Residency Preceptors Conference and one of the six regional residency conferences for residents, fellows, and preceptors.

Pharmacy residencies play an important role in producing clinicians, managers, and leaders for the pharmacy profession. This role has been heightened by changes in the delivery of health care and in the opportunities that are being afforded to pharmacists for drug therapy management and for health promotion and disease prevention activities. Managed care has resulted in a redistribution of patient care from the inpatient to the outpatient setting, which has increased the acuity level of patients in both settings. Pharmacists with more specialized knowledge and training are needed to manage these very complex patients.

Also, health care is slowly transitioning from an illness model to a wellness model with an increasing emphasis being placed on primary, secondary, and tertiary prevention. This requires pharmacists with different skills (e.g., patient risk assessment and behavior modification, immunization delivery, disease screening, and collaborative drug therapy management). Additionally, there have been advances in technology related to pharmaceuticals, information systems, and drug distribution systems. Pharmacists, especially managers, must have a greater understanding of the entire medication management system (drug procurement and storage, prescribing, drug preparation and dispensing, administration, and monitoring), patient safety, continuous quality improvement, population management, and inpatient and outpatient pharmacy operations.

On top of all this, the U.S. population is increasing in diversity (e.g., age, race/ethnicity, country of origin, highest level of education, verbal and written language fluency, economic status), which introduces issues of cultural competency and health literacy into health care. In addition, more and more Americans lack health insurance. Pharmacy residencies can build upon the foundation of knowledge and skills learned in these areas in pharmacy school and properly prepare pharmacists for advanced clinical practice and management roles. Pharmacy residencies also focus on leadership development. Being a good leader is of critical importance whether a pharmacist is a clinical member of a health care team or is a director of a pharmacy department. Completing a pharmacy residency may be the best option for a pharmacist that desires to be a clinical pharmacy specialist or a pharmacy director, especially if he/she wants to work in an academic health system.

Although pharmacy education has been strengthened by conversion from the Bachelor of Science to the Doctor of Pharmacy degree program, pharmacists will still need additional training before being competent to practice in more advanced clinical roles or to manage pharmacy operations. Like the practice of medicine, the practice of pharmacy is becoming more complex and specialized and is requiring more education and training. The exponential increase in medical and pharmaceutical information is making it very hard to be a generalist. As nurse practitioners and physician assistants have taken some of the routine general medical responsibilities from physicians, pharmacy technicians and technology will take some of the routine general pharmacy responsibilities from pharmacists. Ultimately, the health care quality and practitioner competency movements may push regulatory agencies to codify certain requirements and credentials (e.g., residency training, board certification) for pharmacists in advanced practice settings.

Besides being a clinical health care profession focused on providing patient-centered care, pharmacy is also a scientific discipline (the art and science of pharmacy). Advances in the pharmaceutical, clinical, and administrative sciences help propel the pharmacy profession forward. Master of Science and Doctor of Philosophy degree programs have been the traditional source of education and training for research-oriented careers in pharmacy. However, pharmacy fellowships can also prepare pharmacists to conduct research, especially practice-based research (clinical, epidemiological, outcomes). Completing a pharmacy fellowship may be the best option for a pharmacist desiring to be a clinician-scientist and to work at an academic health system for a school of pharmacy or medicine.

Besides being of benefit to their graduates, pharmacy residencies and fellowships can be of benefit to the preceptors, practice sites, and universities. Preceptors can derive a lot of internal satisfaction from training residents and fellows. It helps keep them up-to-date in their fields and allows them to give something back to the pharmacy profession. Additionally, residents and fellows can assist preceptors with their work and expand their capabilities and scope. In the case of patient care activities, this can have a positive impact on the practice site as well. Residents provide significant patient care at a minimum cost. Also, the presence of a residency program can increase the reputation of a pharmacy department both internal and external to the institution. This can create more opportunities for expansion of pharmacy services as well as help with recruitment and retention of pharmacists. Residents and fellows in programs affiliated with pharmacy schools are involved in teaching pharmacy students in didactic, small group problem-based learning, laboratory, and experiential courses. Resident participation as clinical instructors can make a significant contribution to the teaching mission.

As part of personal and professional development planning for their future, all pharmacy students and young pharmacy practitioners should try to define their career goals and aspirations. They should consider whether their goals require that they complete a pharmacy residency or fellowship. If so, they can better position themselves for the initial and subsequent jobs they desire and prepare themselves to make the differences they seek as leaders in pharmacy practice, education, research, management, or service.

References

1. Definitions of pharmacy residencies and fellowships. *Amer J Hosp Pharm.* 1987;44:1142–4.
2. American Society of Health-System Pharmacists. Residency and accreditation information. Available at: http://www.ashp.org.
3. American College of Clinical Pharmacy. Directory of residencies and fellowships. Available at: http://www.accp.com/resandfel/.

I feel that the greatest reward for doing is the opportunity to do more.

Jonas Salk

The Need for Additional Credentials

Kevin Purcell

Objectives

- Discuss the potential reasons for acquiring additional education, training, and credentials.
- Discuss the many options available for working adults to obtain additional education, training, and credentials.

Short-term and long-term career plans should take into consideration the types of education, training, and credentials that will be required or at least helpful in positioning oneself for desired future opportunities. Professional growth and development, lifelong learning, and career advancement necessitate continuous pursuit of new knowledge and skills. This may go beyond what is acquired through attending routine, continuing education programs and engaging in self-directed, independent study. Medical and pharmaceutical information is increasing at an exponential rate. The practice of pharmacy is changing and adapting based on new professional needs. Fortunately, there are many options available for working pharmacists to obtain additional education, training, and credentials, including focused education courses, advanced degrees, skills-based training workshops, and certifications.

Focused education courses are typically offered by a university or by a university working in partnership with a professional society or health care organization (employer). The most visible examples are executive management and leadership courses. These vary in length from intensive weeklong courses to full semester courses delivered during the evenings or on the weekends. This option may be good for pharmacists that want education in a specific area but do not want to invest the time, money, and effort into completing an entire degree program. The weeklong courses do not provide college credit, but the full semester courses usually do, and this credit may possibly be applied to obtaining a degree in the future.

Master's and doctoral degree programs are offered in a variety of fields that may be of benefit to practicing pharmacists, and many universities have master's and doctoral degree programs targeted toward working adults. These can be distance education programs provided either online or through a variety of media or campus-based programs offered during the evenings or on the weekends. Pharmacists commonly obtain master's degrees in hospital pharmacy administration (M.S.), business administration (M.B.A.), health care administration (M.H.A.), and public health (M.P.H.). These credentials may be important when pursuing administrative positions in hospitals and other health care organizations.

Some pharmacists may even decide to obtain a doctoral degree in one of these areas (e.g., Ph.D., D.B.A., D.H.A., or Dr.P.H.), especially if they work in an academic health center and are heavily involved in teaching students, residents, and fellows. Some pharmacists with a primary responsibility for teaching obtain a master's degree (M.Ed.) or a doctoral degree (Ph.D.) in education. This is particularly useful in academia when one is responsible for curriculum development and outcomes assessment, faculty development, distance education programs, and experiential education programs. Of course, many pharmacists have obtained a nontraditional Doctor of Pharmacy degree. These programs have been important for pharmacists transitioning from a drug distribution role to a patient care role. Finally, a few pharmacists go back to graduate school full-time to obtain a doctoral degree in one of the pharmaceutical sciences (Ph.D.) and pursue a research-oriented career track in academia or the pharmaceutical industry. Keep in mind that some employers may pay for their employees to complete master's or doctoral programs if it will better prepare them for their current position or for a future position with the organization.

Skills-based workshops are offered in a variety of clinical areas (e.g., basic clinical skills, physical assessment, anticoagulation, asthma, diabetes, immunizations, and herbals). Skills-based workshops are usually developed by pharmacy professional organizations and pharmacy schools. These skills-based workshops are typically one or two days in length and provide continuing education approved by the Accreditation Council for Pharmacy Education (ACPE). Some of these workshops are linked to certification programs. This option may be good for pharmacists that want focused training in a specific area, especially those looking to expand the scope of their practice. Also, various health care organizations offer skills-based certification courses in basic cardiac life support (BCLS) and advanced cardiac life support (ACLS). These can be useful for anyone in general, especially BCLS, and they are of particular importance in institutions where pharmacists serve as members of the code team.

There are a number of organizations that offer certification exams for pharmacists and other health care professionals. Certification can be a useful credential for pharmacists in a clinical or a management career track. There appears to be increasing recognition and value placed on certification. Certification has been linked in some cases to employment and pay, clinical privileges, provider status on third party payer plans, and reimbursement for services. The Board of Pharmaceutical Specialties (BPS; www.bpsweb.org) offers certification exams in pharmacotherapy, psychiatric pharmacy, nuclear pharmacy, nutrition support pharmacy, and oncology pharmacy. The American Board of Clinical Pharmacology (ABCP; www.abcp.net) offers a certification exam in clinical pharmacology. The American Board of Toxicology (ABT; www.abtox.org) offers a certification exam in toxicology. The American Association of Diabetes Educators (AADE; www.aadenet.org) offers a certification exam in diabetes education. The American College of Healthcare Executives (ACHE; www.ache.org) offers a certification exam in health care management. The National Institute for Standards in Pharmacist Credentialing (NISPC; www.nispcnet.org) offers certification exams in disease state management, including asthma, diabetes, dyslipidemia, and anticoagulation. Pharmacists interested in learning more about certification should visit the websites of these organizations to review the process, requirements, and eligibility criteria.

Life begets life. Energy creates energy. It is by spending oneself that one becomes rich.

Sarah Bernhardt

Chapter 10

Mentors

Debra S. Devereaux, Rita R. Shane

Chapter Outline

The best way to find yourself is to lose yourself in the service of others.

Mahatma Ghandi

Finding the Right Blends in a Mentor-Student Relationship

Rita R. Shane

Objectives

- Recognize traits that are important in order to be an effective mentor.
- Create an environment conducive to mentoring.
- Support the student's development of self-esteem.
- Introduce the student to professionalism.
- Identify qualities in the student that are important for a successful mentor-protégé relationship.
- Recognize the rewards that mentoring offers.

Mentoring has its origin in the story of Odysseus where Athena portrays multiple roles in order to guide Telemachus, Odysseus' son, during Odysseus' journey. One of these roles is that of *Mentor* where Athena serves as "advisor, teacher, sponsor, counselor, coach advocate, and role model."[1] Mentoring is a journey that enables the student or protégé to develop both professionally and personally. This chapter will describe the many roles that mentors play in guiding growth and development and highlight the qualities that are important in both the mentor and the protégé. The terms *student* and *protégé* will be used interchangeably throughout this chapter.

Characteristics of Mentor-Protégé Relationships

Mentor-protégé relationships are developed based on shared values and vision. The mentor should not be assigned but rather needs to be selected by the student or protégé to ensure that the relationship is successful. The protégé needs to examine the background of potential mentors as part of the selection process. Considerations include the following[2]:

- Is the mentor going to support personal or professional development? Or both?
- Have other students had positive experiences with the mentor?
- Has the mentor served as an advocate for students?
- Are the mentor's areas of interest consistent with that of the student?
- What has the mentor achieved in his/her career?
- Will the mentor have time to devote to the relationship?
- Does the mentor have a professional network that will facilitate development of future relationships for the student?
- Will the mentor challenge the student and also be able to provide nurturing?
- Will the mentor create an environment where the student feels at ease to discuss concerns and fears?

Mentor as the Coach and Advisor

Your role as a mentor will take on many forms as the relationship develops. First and foremost is serving as an advisor and coach by providing direction as the student learns about aspects of pharmacy and the profession. As the mentor, your role is to guide the student through his/her learning experience and potential career pathways rather than to directly tell the student what he/she should do. In order to be effective in this role, you must be present in a way that is more than physical. Being present means that you take the time to focus on the protégé and listen without seeming to be preoccupied or distracted with other responsibilities so that the protégé feels comfortable and is able to open up. Creating open communication is essential in order to break down barriers that inevitably exist since the preceptor-student relationship is traditionally perceived by the student as a hierarchy. A key strategy is to demonstrate vulnerability by sharing your personal experiences, including challenges you have experienced, mistakes that you have made, and the lessons that you have learned. As a result of this process, you will build trust with the protégé, and the protégé will feel comfortable sharing his/her feelings with you. This enables you to begin the mentoring process and serve as coach and advisor to the student. Through ongoing open communication, you can help the protégé discover his/her strengths, weaknesses, talents, skills, likes, and dislikes. Your role is also to encourage the protégé to confront challenges and take risks by communicating your support and confidence in the protégé. Eleanor Roosevelt stated, "You must do the things you think you cannot do."[1] As a mentor, you play an essential role in helping the protégé develop confidence and self-esteem.

Mentor as the Guide and Host

As a mentor, you also serve as a host and guide by introducing the student to individuals within the field of pharmacy and to other health care professionals within your own organization. This enables the student to see how different aspects of pharmacy come together and the key role that pharmacists play in ensuring the safety of the medication use process. As a result, the protégé may meet new potential mentors who can serve as role models both now and in the future. As host, your role is also to introduce the student to pharmacy professional organizations and opportunities for getting involved in the profession, networking, and learning about different career options. If you are able to actually attend a professional meeting with the student, you will have the opportunity to show the student how to network with others in the profession. Your role as guide is to enable the student to discover the many possibilities within pharmacy. Through this process, you will support the protégé's development of a sense of pride in becoming a pharmacist and the motivation to become involved in the profession.

Mentor as the Role Model

The mentor also serves as a role model who, besides possessing a strong knowledge base, demonstrates caring, passion, a sense of humor, and integrity. Caring and compassion are important aspects of every human relationship and even more so in creating a bond between yourself and the student. It is important to remember that these qualities may appear to be absent during busy times or when external factors are creating a stressful situation for you. Communicating to the student that you are preoccupied with something—without necessarily having to share specifics—is important so that the student recognizes something else is going on. This acknowledgement also shows the student, by example, the importance of communication about factors impacting the quality of one's interactions with others. The ideal mentor is passionate about pharmacy and the many opportunities that pharmacists have to demonstrate value by improving management of chronic diseases, preventing medication errors, and serving as a resource to other health care professionals and patients. When asked what an important quality of a mentor is, the protégés will usually list a sense of humor since it makes them feel more comfortable and contributes to a positive mentor-protégé relationship.

Values are of particular importance in the pharmacy profession because of the key role we play in patient safety. It is important to discuss values with the student since it is not uncommon for these values to be tested as patient care issues arise. Examples of situations where value issues are involved: an order for a medication where there is insufficient data regarding efficacy and a potential concern about safety; an expensive drug ordered in a patient without insurance coverage; and a mandate to reduce expenses, which would result in staffing reductions and jeopardize patient safety. Having discussions about value conflicts is an important contributor to the protégé's growth and understanding of how to deal with difficult issues. Finally, mentors play an important role in introducing students to the importance of—and the satisfaction that comes with—being committed to lifelong learning. This is shown by sharing recent articles from the scientific or health care literature with the student and taking time to discuss some of the key points that were addressed.

Protégé Prerequisites

In order for the relationship to be successful, there are a number of prerequisites for the protégé.[3] The protégé needs to be *mentorable*, which means possessing qualities such as intellectual curiosity, initiative, motivation, and follow-through. The mentor must be *present* in order for the experience to be effective, and the protégé must be *ready* by showing interest in communicating with you and asking for guidance. In many ways, the protégé's commitment to the relationship is very similar to that of the mentor; the protégé needs to invest the time, share experiences, and engage in open and honest dialogue. The protégé also needs to follow through on tasks or recommendations; otherwise you will feel that the relationship is not reciprocal.[2] However, even more essential is the protégé's readiness to be open to learn. One could argue here that if the mentor is right, the protégé is ready. This is true; however, sometimes even though the mentor and student are seemingly compatible, the student has too many other priorities or is not yet at a stage of maturity where he/she is ready to be mentored.

Mentor-Protégé Relationship

The mentoring protégé relationship is a reciprocal one in that both individuals experience growth and self-discovery. In the traditional mentoring model, the mentor helps the protégé to develop and the relationship is more equal (Figure 10-1).

A new mentoring paradigm has been suggested in which the relationship evolves such that what begins with the mentor serving as coach and advisor to the protégé becomes a 360 degree process as depicted in the figure below.[4] The relationship begins with the mentor serving as counselor to the protégé. In the next phase (Phase 2), the mentor and protégé become equals as the protégé develops into a professional. This is followed by the protégé serving as a counselor to the mentor, and in this phase (Phase 3), it is the former mentor who learns from the protégé. Lastly, the protégé becomes the mentor, and the process begins again with a new protégé (Phase 4) (Figure 10-2).

In summary, the mentor-protégé relationship is one where both the "heart and the mind" are nurtured.[1] The quality of the interaction is based on mutual respect, openness, and honesty. The mentor guides students by weaving together their strengths, weaknesses, likes, and dislikes and helps students

Figure 10-1. Traditional Mentoring Model

Mentor (M) ⇒Protégé (P).

Figure 10-2. New Mentoring Paradigm[4]

	Phase 1	Phase 2	Phase 3	Phase 4
M ⇒	Mp ⇒	MP ⇒	mP ⇒	P

(P returns to M: ↑ ← ↓)

discover themselves. The mentor serves as advisor, counselor, coach, therapist, guide, and companion. The growth experienced in this relationship is mutual, and it is the reciprocity in the relationship that makes it fulfilling for both.

References

1. Wilthire SF. *Athena's Disguises: Mentors in Everyday Life.* Louisville: Westminster John Knox Press; 1998.
2. Hoffman B. Mentoring: on having one and being one. ACCP. http://www.aacp.org/site/tertiary.asp?TRACKID=&VID=2&CID=513&DID=3939. Accessed January 29, 2004.
3. APEGGA. Mentoring: attributes of a receptive protégé. http://www.apegga.org/publications/guidelines/mentor/protege.htm. Accessed January 29, 2004.
4. Gray WA. What is the new mentoring paradigm? www.mentoring-resources.com. Accessed May 12, 1999.

Every great man is always being helped by everybody; for his gift is to get good out of all things and persons.

John Ruskin

Comparison of Skills and Characteristics of Precepting vs. Mentoring

Debra S. Devereaux

Objectives

- Compare the characteristics of a preceptor relationship versus a mentoring relationship.
- Identify the traits that constitute a mentor-protégé pairing.
- Recognize behaviors that detract from a mentor-protégé relationship.
- Reflect on the personal and professional challenges of being a mentor.
- Affirm the rewards of a successful mentoring process.

By the time we are adults, most of us can identify people who have had a significant influence on our learning and development in our professional life and/or our personal life. For hundreds of years, mentoring has been used as a method for handing down knowledge, maintaining culture, supporting talent, and securing future leadership.[1] Research indicates the mentoring process is linked to career success, personal growth, and increased organizational productivity.

Comparison of the Preceptor Relationship and the Mentoring Relationship

The precepting relationship is associated with student learning experiences. It has a defined beginning and ending. Students may have requested the site and the preceptor voluntarily, or they may have been assigned to that site involuntarily. There are specific learning objectives and tasks that students must achieve during the experiential rotation.

The State of California's Pharmacy Intern Preceptor Manual states "Specific activities are planned that will contribute to the mastery of each task and practice responsibility. These might include: daily practice responsibilities, observation of selected tasks, special assignments and projects, reading journal articles or other references, attending meetings and seminars and discussions with the intern and other pharmacists."[2] For example, a typical six-week-rotation at an ambulatory care clinic might include taking patient medication histories, evaluating laboratory values, monitoring medication levels, titrating patient medications, participating in journal club, physical assessment, and patient counseling. Students are formally evaluated by the preceptor on their mastery and completion of the rotation objectives. Students evaluate the precepted site and the preceptor based on their experience.

In a formal mentoring program, a mentee or protégé may be assigned a mentor. Formal mentoring models are authoritarian because they are introduced and controlled by a senior manager. This model normally occurs in a work environment where a new employee is assigned to be "shown the ropes" by a senior employee or an employee with more experience. A formal mentoring relationship also usually has a defined duration. At the end of six months or one year, the formal reporting requirements and amount of time required to be spent together ends. In this way, a precepted rotation is an example of a formal mentoring program. Some of the objectives can even be the same such as indoctrination to the organization culture, department protocol, and the transferring of knowledge. A precepting relationship may evolve into a mentoring relationship when both the preceptor and the student desire to continue their collaboration.

MENTOR PEARLS

A mentor's role is to "hold the mirror" for protégés. A mentor asks questions rather than giving answers.

How mentoring is defined and used appears to depend on the participant's point of view. However, there is much more to mentoring than giving advice. The Webster dictionary definition of mentor is "a trusted counselor or guide; tutor; coach." Formal mentoring programs became more prevalent in the 1970s in business and government agencies. In the 1980s, school districts and universities picked up on the idea for their teachers.

Goals and Benefits of Mentoring to the Protégé (Mentee) and the Mentor

Transformation

In a successful mentoring relationship both you, as the mentor, and the protégé should be changed by your experiences. You may have helped the protégé to uncover an aspect, ability, or talent that had either lain dormant or gone unrecognized. The protégé may be inspired to shift the direction of his/her life in a constructive way. The protégé may have caused you to question long held beliefs and gain new understanding or a new outlook.

Reciprocity or Mutuality

For your mentoring relationship to be effective, both of you must perceive benefits. The protégé and you need to feel that the time you have spent together has been valuable. Both of you need to feel mutual respect. Communication lines must be open and travel in both directions. Your relationship should be a win-win situation for both parties.

MENTOR PEARLS

A mentor is not a person with the answers.

Mentor Regeneration

As a result of the mentoring experience, you should feel a sense of renewal and rejuvenation in being a pharmacist. You may feel both personal and professional satisfaction for making a significant contribution to the profession and your organization.

Protégé Moves toward Being a Peer

Studies have shown that protégés in successful mentoring relationships have a positive attitude toward their work and perceive less stress than individuals without a mentor. A dynamic mentoring relationship allows the protégé to grow and eventually become an equal of yours and go on to be a mentor to others.

Sharing and Challenging

As a mentor you need to be willing to share your knowledge and experience. You may provide suggestions and advice in the form of "If I was in your position," or "Here's something you might consider," or "Whatever you think will work best, you do." You should utilize tutoring methods, which rely on asking questions and asking for plans. You should encourage your protégé to brainstorm—there are no bad ideas.

MENTOR PEARLS

Focus on wisdom. Be a resource, catalyst, facilitator, idea generator, networker, or problem-solver.

Pitfalls and Challenges of Mentoring

Protégés need feedback, evaluation, and challenge. You, as a mentor, need to strike a balance between support and stretching beyond the protégé's abilities.

You should try not to point out the right and wrong of what a protégé does rather than getting at the thought process that led to the decision. You are interested in the *why* of the protégé's thinking rather than trying to fix it for him or her.

MENTOR PEARLS

Be patient. Don't rush into the silence. Silence is a stimulator.

The protégé should challenge your thinking. Why did you decide to become a pharmacist; What was it like starting out; and How did you deal with challenges in your work or personal life?

You and the protégé should avoid boundary violations: gift giving, finding the protégé a new job or promotion, loaning money, and sexual flirtation are out-of-bounds in a mentoring relationship.

A mentoring relationship can endure two to five years or last a lifetime. There are natural ebbs and flows where one or the other person is more invested in the

MENTOR PEARLS

Experiment with process. Use coaching, role playing, simulations, brainstorming, or try a change of scenery by going for a walk together or attending a sporting event.

relationship, and there are different mentoring needs as a person progresses through life.

It is essential that privacy, honesty, and integrity be maintained in your mentoring relationship. What is said in the relationship is confidential.

MENTOR PEARLS

The amount of time spent listening should be at least four times the amount spent talking.

In the most rewarding mentoring relationships, you and the protégé have mutually identified each other. You may see the protégé as a younger version of yourself. The protégé may see you as a role model. However, the key to a successful match is not how similar you and the protégé are. Ideally, you will be able to provide just the right help to the protégé at just the right time. You are holding up the mirror for the protégé's future pharmacy career.

References

1. Darwin A. Critical reflections on mentoring in work settings. *Adult Education Quarterly*. 2002;50(3):197–211.
2. California State Board of Pharmacy. *Intern Preceptor Manual*. http://www.pharmacy.ca.gov/intern_preceptor_manual.htm. Accessed January 18, 2004.
3. Wright S, Smith D. A case for formalized mentoring. *Quest*. 2000;52:200–13.
4. Tips for Mentors. http://mentors.ca/mentorideas.htm. Accessed March 2002.

If I can dream, I can act and if I can act, I can become.

Poh Yu Khing

Chapter 11

Professionalism and Professional Socialization

David Lorms, John E. Murphy, Kevin Purcell

Chapter Outline

Success in the end erases all the mistakes along the way.

Chinese Proverb

Professionalism

Kevin Purcell

Objectives

- Explain what it means to *be* a pharmacist.
- Define professionalism and professionalization.
- Describe how to influence a student's professional perspective and development over time and through activities and environment.
- Explain the importance of setting clear expectations regarding professionalism.

"Before one can do what a pharmacist does, one must know how to be what a pharmacist is. The practice of pharmacy is not about dispensing drugs, but about taking care of patients."[1]

Being a pharmacist goes far beyond merely graduating from pharmacy school, passing the NAPLEX and MPJE, and having an active pharmacy license. By the same token, being a professional goes far beyond merely becoming a member of a profession. Certainly, pharmacists do dispense drugs, but our higher purpose and calling as health care professionals is to take care of patients. Pharmacists help patients and their physicians with the management of the patient's drug therapy and overall health. A pharmacist must understand what it means to be a health care professional before he/she can successfully serve that higher purpose and calling. The concept of being a pharmacist ultimately refers to the embodiment of all the hallmark qualities and characteristics (e.g., commitment, self-sacrifice, pride, knowledge, skills, abilities, values, attitudes, beliefs, and behaviors) of a pharmacy professional. A profession is defined as an occupation whose members share 10 common characteristics (Figure 11-1).[2] A professional is defined as a member of a profession who displays 10 common traits (Figure 11-2).[2] Professionalism is then the active demonstration of the traits of a professional.[2] Finally, professionalization (professional socialization)

Figure 11-1 • Definition of a Profession*

Profession: An occupation whose members share 10 common characteristics.

1. Prolonged specialized training in a body of abstract knowledge
2. A service orientation
3. An ideology based on the original faith professed by members
4. An ethic that is binding on the practitioners
5. A body of knowledge unique to the members
6. A set of skills that forms the technique of the profession
7. A guild of those entitled to practice the profession
8. Authority granted by society in the form of licensure and certification
9. A recognized setting where the profession is practiced
10. A theory of societal benefits derived from the ideology

*Developed by the American Pharmaceutical Association Academy of Students of Pharmacy and the American Association of Colleges of Pharmacy Council of Deans Task Force on Professionalism.

Figure 11-2 • Definition of a Professional*

Professional: A member of a profession who displays the following 10 traits.

1. Knowledge and skills of a profession
2. Commitment to self-improvement of skills and knowledge
3. Service orientation
4. Pride in the profession
5. Covenantal relationship with the client
6. Creativity and innovation
7. Conscience and trustworthiness
8. Accountability for his/her work
9. Ethically sound decision making
10. Leadership

*Developed by the American Pharmaceutical Association Academy of Students of Pharmacy and the American Association of Colleges of Pharmacy Council of Deans Task Force on Professionalism.

is the process of inculcating a profession's attitudes, values, and behaviors into a professional.[2]

Professionalization of students requires a spectrum of activities over a long period of time in a diverse set of environments (e.g., classroom, practice sites, professional societies, and community service organizations) that positively influence their professional perspective and development. Many people are co-responsible for the professionalization process, including students, faculty, and practitioners, as well as school administrative staff, pharmacy technicians, and other health care professionals.[3] Preceptors need to recognize and appreciate the important role that they play in the professionalization process. Preceptors can have a profound impact on the professionalization of students through role modeling and establishing mentoring relationships.[2,3]

Preceptors may facilitate a discussion on the topic of professionalism with students in a variety of ways and stimulate them to engage in a process of self-assessment, self-reflection, and self-transformation. Preceptors can point out both positive and negative examples of professionalism in patient care, pharmacy operations, and professional and business relationships. Case studies and role-playing exercises may be used to supplement real life situations that occur during the internship. Preceptors can share their thoughts and feelings on professionalism and some of their personal experiences with their own professionalization process. Preceptors can also discuss with students what they do to continue to grow and develop as pharmacy practitioners and health professionals and to attain a level of excellence as patient care providers, teachers, researchers, managers, and/or leaders. Lastly, preceptors can express their professional pride they have about being pharmacists and what it has meant to them—the relationships they have formed with patients and colleagues, the care they have provided, and the difference they have made in people's lives. There is nothing like a true hero story to reinforce the desired pharmacy culture, set a high bar of achievement, and inspire others to outdo what has been done and raise the bar even higher.

There are several important documents that preceptors can use to facilitate a discussion of professionalism and to reinforce professional ideals. The Pledge of Professionalism (Figure 11-3) is often recited by pharmacy students at a

Figure 11-3 • Pledge of Professionalism*

As a student of pharmacy, I believe there is a need to build and reinforce a professional identity founded on integrity, ethical behavior, and honor. This development, a vital process in my education, will help ensure that I am true to the professional relationship I establish between myself and society as I become a member of the pharmacy community. Integrity must be an essential part of my everyday life, and I must practice pharmacy with honesty and commitment to service.

To accomplish this goal of professional development, I, as a student of pharmacy, should adhere to the following:

***DEVELOP** a sense of loyalty and duty to the profession of pharmacy by being a builder of community, one able and willing to contribute to the well-being of others and one who enthusiastically accepts the responsibility and accountability for membership in the profession.*

***FOSTER** professional competency through lifelong learning. I must strive for high ideals, teamwork, and unity within the profession in order to provide optimal patient care.*

***SUPPORT** my colleagues by actively encouraging personal commitment to the Oath of Maimonides and a Code of Ethics as set forth by the profession.*

***INCORPORATE** into my life and practice, dedication to excellence. This will require an ongoing reassessment of personal and professional values.*

***MAINTAIN** the highest ideals and professional attributes to ensure and facilitate the covenantal relationship required of the pharmaceutical caregiver.*

The profession of pharmacy is one that demands adherence to a set of rigid, ethical standards. These high ideals are necessary to ensure the quality of care extended to the patients I serve. As a student of pharmacy, I believe this does not start with graduation; rather, it begins with my membership in this professional college community. Therefore, I must strive to uphold these standards as I advance toward full membership in the profession of pharmacy.

---

*Developed and adopted by the American Pharmaceutical Association Academy of Students of Pharmacy and the American Association of Colleges of Pharmacy Council of Deans Task Force on Professionalism, June 26, 1994.

white coat ceremony during their first professional year. The Oath of a Pharmacist (Figure 11-4) is often recited by pharmacy students at their graduation ceremony. The Code of Ethics for Pharmacists (see chapter 3) states the principles that form the fundamental basis of the roles and responsibilities of pharmacists. Pharmacy students should be familiar with and adhere to all of these critical works that define what it means to be a pharmacist and a health care professional. All provide guidance to those on a lifelong journey to become the best pharmacists they can be. These documents may not encompass everything that one should know about pharmacy professionalism, but they do include reference to all of the key elements of professionalism, including honor/integrity, altruism/advocacy, duty/service, responsibility/accountability, respect for others, compassion/empathy, communication/collaboration, self-awareness/knowledge of limits, and a commitment to lifelong learning and professional growth and development.[4,5] Additionally, preceptors can discuss with students the importance of a positive attitude, professional attire and

Figure 11-4 • OATH OF A PHARMACIST*

At this time, I vow to devote my professional life to the service of all humankind through the profession of pharmacy.

I will consider the welfare of humanity and relief of human suffering my primary concerns.

I will apply my knowledge, experience, and skills to the best of my ability to assure optimal drug therapy outcomes for the patients I serve.

I will keep abreast of developments and maintain professional competency in my profession of pharmacy.

I will maintain the highest principles of moral, ethical, and legal conduct.

I will embrace and advocate change in the profession of pharmacy that improves patient care.

I take these vows voluntarily with the full realization of the responsibility with which I am entrusted by the public.

---

*Developed by the American Pharmaceutical Association Academy of Students of Pharmacy/American Association of Colleges of Pharmacy Council of Deans (APhA-ASP/AACP-COD) Task Force on Professionalism; June 26, 1994.

appearance, punctuality, organization, time management, follow-through, and openness to constructive criticism.

Preceptors need to set clear expectations regarding professionalism at the beginning of the internship. A discussion of professional expectations and examples of intolerable behaviors can be included in the orientation session. Preceptors should also provide periodic formative feedback on the professionalism of students throughout the internship. Optimally, preceptors will have the ability to formally assess the professionalism of students as part of the summative evaluation at the end of the internship. Students should also have the opportunity to assess their own professionalism as part of the evaluation process. Then, if there is a discrepancy between the preceptors' rating and the students' self-evaluation, preceptors can have a final discussion on professionalism with students that examines the difference in their perspectives and stimulates deeper reflection on the part of the students.

Getting to know and working with others are good ways for students to enhance their professionalization and their understanding of the role of pharmacists in the health care system and the community. Communication with patients is absolutely necessary for most internships. Students need to learn how to develop pharmacist-patient relationships based on mutual trust, respect, and commitment. Also, spending time with other health care professionals, either one-on-one or as part of a patient care team, can be very beneficial. Preceptors can take students along and get them involved in any community service or professional society activities in which the preceptors participate. Community service activities can provide students with a broader understanding of issues faced and enhance their cultural competency. Professional society activities can increase student identification with the pharmacy profession and provide students with a network of peers.

Teaching pharmacy students about the important principles of the pharmacy profession and showing students how to live them is a critical responsibility of preceptors. Keep in mind, the messenger is often more important than the message. The messenger must personify the message so the two are in harmony or students will become cynical. Preceptors need to lead by example and create an atmosphere that promotes professionalism, fosters lifelong learning, and nurtures professional growth and development. This can be challenging at times in some practice settings due to work-related and marketplace factors, as well as to general societal influences. It requires a team effort to maintain a professional image and practice environment in any pharmacy setting. Pharmacists, technicians, and students are all part of that team and contribute to establishing and maintaining a climate of professionalism.

References

1. Purcell K. Pharmacy leadership survey: developing pharmacy leaders. *Texas Society of Health-System Pharmacists Journal. 2004;5(2):8–15.*
2. American Pharmaceutical Association Academy of Students of Pharmacy and American Association of Colleges of Pharmacy Council of Deans Task Force on Professionalism. White paper on pharmacy student professionalism. *J Am Pharm Assoc.* 2000;40:96–102.
3. Hammer DP, Berger BA, Beardsley RS, et al. Student professionalism. *Am J Pharm Educ.* 2003;67:Article 96.
4. American Board of Internal Medicine Committee on Evaluation of Clinical Competence and the Clinical Competence and Communication Programs. *Project Professionalism.* Philadelphia, PA: American Board of Internal Medicine; 2001:4–6.
5. Klein EJ, Jackson C, Kratz L, et al. Teaching professionalism to residents. *Acad Med.* 2003;78:26–34.

Treat people as if they were what they ought to be and you help them to become what they are capable of being.

Johann Wolfgang von Goethe

The Role of Participation in Pharmacy Professional Organizations

John E. Murphy

Objectives

- Understand the importance of both preceptor and student involvement in professional pharmacy organizations.
- Describe preceptor modeling as a way to encourage student participation in professional pharmacy organizations.

Importance of Involvement—Preceptors

It is hard to argue that a profession can get along well without leaders, though "leaving it up to someone else" is the most often noted outcome when it comes time to volunteer for leadership opportunities. The 20:80 rule (20% of the people will do 80% of the work) certainly seems to apply in many professional organizations. However, preceptors may not rest among the silent majority when it comes to participation in professional pharmacy organizations. They have accepted positions as role models who inculcate "professional attitudes, ethics, and behaviors."[1] Preceptors are already among the 20% making things happen for the future of the profession when it comes to education. Since students will mimic the behaviors of those people they identify as successful, it is up to you to provide the model of a successful practitioner and leader of the profession, no matter what your job role in the profession might be.

It is, therefore, quite fortunate that participating in professional organizations can add so much to your career as a pharmacist and preceptor role model. For example, through all my years of participating in pharmacy organizations, I cannot recall one volunteer effort that was not at least as beneficial to me personally or professionally as the benefit I provided to the organization. In the past I even commented that these opportunities were nearly akin to thievery.[2]

The notion of gaining from activities outside of traditional studying, such as active participation in organizations, is well known in academia.[3–5] It has been estimated that much of the cognitive development of college students comes from their activities *outside the classroom*.[4] An example of this is the opportunity to discuss issues and academics during dormitory life that leads to enhanced cognitive understanding, much like the opportunities that occur from meeting with colleagues at a professional meeting. Further, participation in student organizations has been specifically identified as playing an integral role in the educational process.[5]

I believe it to be quite reasonable to assume that an important component of your development as a professionally competent clinician, manager, educator, business person, and preceptor also comes, to a significant degree, from activities outside of the daily practice as a pharmacist. Participation in the activities of a professional organization can be one of the great ways to help continue the development of many important job and life skills. The profession needs people who are dedicated to advancing its causes, and you have already made the important commitment to create future generations of colleagues.

So what does *participation* mean for the preceptor? I believe there is a hierarchy but that many of the elements can occur at the same time. Below are activities you should consider in the development of your role as preceptor so you can be the best role model for your students.

- Join the organization and pay dues (critically important as member numbers allow the organization to have a voice).
- Attend meetings and make your voice heard.
- Volunteer for committees/task forces/special projects.
- Chair committees.
- Participate in legislative activities.
- Give presentations and present posters.
- Run for office.

Active participation can generate benefits for you that may then be demonstrated to the students. This allows the profession to benefit now and in the future.

Importance of Involvement—Students

As might be expected, many of the reasons students should begin getting involved in professional organizations during their college years (and certainly after graduation) are the same as those for preceptors. For one, involved students are more likely to see the value of the profession to them and the importance of promoting the profession for their own future. Other important reasons:

- Enhancing professionalism
- Developing future leaders
- Developing an attitude of interest in the profession
- Promoting community service
- Instilling a feeling of obligation to the profession
- Establishing esprit de corps among members of the organizations

Many students will come to their experiential education settings with a wealth of experience in student organizations and college governance.[6] However, it is quite common for those students who were active in student organizations to fall by the wayside once they become practicing professionals.

◆ **Preceptor Pearls**

There are many opportunities for preceptors to get or keep students interested and involved in professional organizations. You are in a critical position to actively mentor students on the value of participation. You can help students see the importance of continuing their involvement if they have been active as students, or you can demonstrate to previously inactive students why it is critical that they now begin participating. Research has shown that faculty, including preceptor faculty, can make a difference in whether a student decides to join a professional organization.[7,8] Thus, taking the time—to not only participate yourself but also to share the reasons why participation in professional organizations is so important for the future of the profession—can provide a strong influence to students under your care and guidance.

The professional organizations understand this phenomenon and work very hard to attract graduates to their fold with programs such as Young Practitioners and with reduced dues for the first year. Unfortunately, these incentives are only partially effective, thus creating opportunities for preceptors to reinforce the value of participation in professional organizations.

Selected Modeling Suggestions

- Discuss the value of participating in a professional organization with students.
- Invite your students to a local professional meeting, or even better, take them with you.
- If feasible, make it a rotation requirement that students attend at least one meeting in a professional organization and report back to you on what occurred during the meeting.
- Introduce students to influential pharmacists and potential employers at a meeting.
- Have the students recognized as new attendees during a meeting.
- Bring the students to a committee meeting.
- Help the students get on a committee.
- Sponsor students. Pay part of the students' attendance fee at a pharmacy meeting or part of their dues to a professional organization. Even a small part demonstrates clear commitment on your part. Tell them why you are providing the sponsorship. Encourage other pharmacists to participate in Sponsor a Student programs.

Didactic Opportunities

- Conduct a study session on a professional organization. Have the students compare and contrast selected national organizations (mission, vision, services).
- Discuss the reasons why people join organizations (the general reasons, and then personalize your situation).
- Assign readings and discuss the history of various organizations such as the American Society of Health-System Pharmacists[9] and the American

Pharmacists Association (articles are printed in most issues of the *Journal of the American Pharmacists Association*).

- Give the students a sense of the profession's leaders (e.g., read and discuss the Harvey A.K. Whitney Award Lectures[10] or articles about individual leaders).[11]
- Discuss international pharmacy organizations (e.g., The International Pharmaceutical Federation at FIP, http://www.fip.org/) and how pharmacy in other countries may affect practice in the United States.

These are only a few of the many reasons why it is important for preceptors and students to be involved in professional organizations and why you can make a difference in the lives of students when it comes to advancing the profession. You have already made an extremely important contribution to the future of our profession by serving as a preceptor. Participating in professional organizations allows you to continue to grow personally as a professional and allows many opportunities to inspire students and to model what is needed in our future generations of pharmacists.

References

1. Accreditation Council for Pharmacy Education—*Accreditation Standards, Guideline 11.6*. http://www.acpe-accredit.org/standards/standards1.asp.
2. Murphy JE. Confessions of a pharmacy thief. *Am J Health-Syst Pharm*. 1996;53:2522–3.
3. Pascarella ER, Terenzini PT. *How College Affects Students: Findings and Insights from Twenty Years of Research*. San Francisco: Jossey-Bass Publishers; 1991.
4. Kuh GD. The other curriculum: out-of-class experiences associated with student learning and personal development. *J Higher Educ*. 1995;66(2):123–55.
5. Miller TK, Jones JD. Out-of-class activities. In: Chickering AW, et al. *The Modern American College: Responding to the New Realities of Diverse Students and a Changing Society*. San Francisco: Jossey-Bass Publishers; 1981:657–71.
6. Cox ER, Krueger KP, Murphy JE. Pharmacy student involvement in student organizations. *J Pharm Teaching*. 1998;6:9–18.
7. Slack MK, Murphy JE. Faculty influence and other factors associated with student membership in professional organizations. *Am J Pharm Educ*. 1995;59:125–30.
8. Murphy JE, Slack MK. Pharmacy students: the link to our future—Guidelines to increase student participation in professional organizations. Bethesda, MD: American Society of Hospital Pharmacists; 1993.
9. Harris RR, McConnell WE. The American Society of Hospital Pharmacists: a history. *Am J Hosp Pharm*. 1993;50(suppl 2):S1–S45.

10. Harvey AK. Whitney Award Lectures (1950–2003). Bethesda, MD: ASHP Research and Education Foundation; 2004.
11. Worthen DB. Joseph Price Remington (1847–1918). *J Am Pharm Assoc.* 2002;42(4):664–6.

Volunteer service is the rent we pay to our community.

Anonymous

Community Service: The Broader Role of Professionalism

David Lorms

Objectives

- Describe how to help students identify professional skills that can be developed through community service activities.
- Explain how involvement can broaden students' understanding of professional organization opportunities.
- Describe a process for students to determine their own community service interest areas.

Other parts of this handbook have addressed the various roles of the preceptor in direct relationship to the students under their tutelage and the practice of pharmacy. By addressing professionalism and professional socialization, this chapter recognizes an underappreciated but essential overarching aspect of the pharmacist in society.

As much as pharmacists play an important role in public health policy and its implementation and development, it is imperative that students see themselves actively engaged in this important role. Regardless of their practice site, pharmacy as a profession—through the involvement of its individual practitioners—has been instrumental in its support for a variety of public health issues at the local level. For the rent to our communities to be continually marked *paid,* an important responsibility you have as a preceptor is to ensure students have a broad exposure and see themselves as integral to the success of volunteer service of any sort.

My first association position in New Mexico exposed me to pharmacists active in their respective community, using their individual talents to move forward the agenda of a state component of a national health association. One of these provided essential linkages to different connections to the community previously inaccessible to those in formal leadership positions. The second, through his role as a state representative, provided guidance to this group in the ways of legislation and political connection.

To be certain, students will not have this depth of capacity to offer as they come directly from school; however, they should be led by you to find their own respective niche in the world of volunteerism—a niche that they might be able to grow with as they progress in the profession.

Tom Peters, in his treatise *The Brand You 50*, suggests that one can assume responsibilities for many of those smaller, less glamorous tasks in organizations and turn them into success steps in your career.[1] These tasks can be found in churches, almost any nationally focused health agency, or the public school system as Phil Johnson, a past president of the Florida Society of Health-System Pharmacists, found. Johnson uncovered a simple truth that the school systems are a large provider of health care to our children. Today he is the chief volunteer leader for a nationally known and respected program that FSHP sponsors called Medication Use in Schools.

In the current vernacular, "What's in it for me?" has significant weight for volunteerism. Students must be shown how the pay for volunteer work translates into a sense of accomplishment and feeling of achievement and how the exposure to new audiences (or activities) can engage their spirit and provide recognition. Then essential threads in the warp and woof of the communities in our professional and public lives will be weakened.

Students' appreciation for their time and effort can be engaged by illustrating how their skills in communications, facilitation, planning, speaking, writing, or delegating (when paired with characteristics of accessibility, team play, goal-orientation, vision, sense of success, and personal commitment to a cause) can indeed make a significant and positive impact on *their* community.

Pointing students to opportunities of interest should be easy. It is important to help them see a personal stake in their first few ventures to ensure the experience is a positive and profound one. Aside from the major health agencies, smaller community groups also need assistance. As a preceptor you should also consider focusing their interest as it warrants to the political process for both state and federal elections. This last group of opportunities will undoubtedly open their eyes to further interest in societal environmental factors that impact their profession.

Student interest should be directed to professional organizations as well. No matter the students' practice interest, there are at least one or two organizations to support their short- and long-term professional development. It is these groups where their professional commitment can be hardened, preparing them for a career rich in professional connections and community.

Reference

1. Peters, T. *The Brand You 50: Fifty Ways to Transform Yourself from an 'Employee' into a Brand That Shouts Distinction, Commitment, and Passion!* New York: Alfred A. Knopf, Inc.; 1999.

Nothing great was ever achieved without enthusiasm.

Ralph Waldo Emerson

Pharmacy Spirit

Kevin Purcell

Objectives

- Define pharmacy spirit as it relates to forming good pharmacist-patient relationships, effectively practicing the art and science of pharmacy, and continuously improving patient care and advancing the pharmacy profession.
- Describe how preceptors can be role models for students, lead by example, and display pharmacy spiriting and embody its elements.
- Describe how preceptors can get students to exhibit pharmacy spirit.

"Pharmacy spirit is the energy, loyalty, dedication, and courage that push forward the frontiers of pharmacy practice. Pharmacy spirit is the heart and driving force behind providing and improving patient care. Pharmacy spirit is the enthusiasm, determination, and commitment, as well as the love, compassion, and kindness required for providing the best possible patient care. It is the soul of the pharmacy profession. Having pharmacy spirit symbolizes the ultimate commitment to the pharmacy oath, and therefore to the profession of pharmacy and to the public."[1,2]

Pharmacy spirit describes the humanistic qualities, character, and strong will that are necessary to form good patient-pharmacist relationships, effectively practice the art and science of pharmacy, and continuously improve patient care and advance the pharmacy profession. It is the force of this spirit that all outstanding pharmacy practitioners and leaders feel and draw on. Having pharmacy spirit gives meaning to the practice of pharmacy by putting into broader context the little things that are done as part of routine daily work, which make a difference in the lives of others. Instilling pharmacy spirit into students is the culmination of precepting and mentoring. Exemplary preceptors and mentors radiate pharmacy spirit and energize their preceptees and mentees to be the best pharmacists they can be and to make a positive impact on the lives of the people they serve. Having and radiating pharmacy spirit and instilling pharmacy spirit into others may be the quintessential expression of pharmacy professionalism. Ultimately, when students fully appreciate and use the power of pharmacy spirit, the torch of leadership is passed from one generation to the next. Leadership is central to the concept of pharmacy spirit. Power as it relates to pharmacy spirit is no different from power as it relates to positive thinking. In both cases, your inspiration and success come from a mindset and a way of thinking and viewing the world.

Role Models

By demonstrating a commitment to the Oath of a Pharmacist and the Code of Ethics for Pharmacists and through their actions with patients and other health-care professionals, the preceptor becomes a role model. As role models for students, preceptors must lead by example and display pharmacy spirit and embody its elements (Figure 11-5). Preceptors can show care and respect for others by having compassion and sensitivity and helping them maintain their dignity and self-esteem. Preceptors can demonstrate pharmacy spirit by putting the needs of patients first and by understanding the impact of their actions and others on their patients. Preceptors can demonstrate how to take action and assume responsibility for the care of patients by being alert, having a high index of suspicion, and resolving any actual or potential drug-related problems and any other health care-related issues that are identified and could adversely affect patient outcomes. Preceptors can display a drive to achieve excellence as practitioners by trying out new ways of doing things in order to advance the practice of pharmacy and improve patient care. Preceptors can discuss with students the need to renew and reinvent themselves through a continual process of self-assessment, self-reflection, and self-transformation. Preceptors can talk with students about the history of their profession, important pharmacy traditions, and distinguished pharmacists who led the way in the past. Above all, preceptors must have a passion for what they do, a positive attitude, and a true desire to serve the public and to help students grow and develop.

Ultimately, preceptors want their students to posses and exhibit pharmacy

Figure 11-5 • The Elements of Pharmacy Spirit

P rofessionalism
H eart
A ction
R enewal
M entoring
A dventure
C aring
Y earning

S ervice
P assion
I deals
R esponsibility
I magination
T radition

spirit. Preceptors can encourage their students and acknowledge and praise them when they demonstrate their ability to help advance the practice of pharmacy and improve patient care. People have a tendency to rise to the level of expectation and belief that others have in them (the Pygmalion effect). Preceptors can talk with students about each other's experiences with patient care, pharmacy practice, and leadership and stimulate reflective thinking and learning about what it means to be a pharmacist, a health care professional, and a leader. Finally, preceptors can recognize and reward their students when they show pharmacy spirit. For example, preceptors could present a pharmacy spirit certificate to students who radiate and exemplify pharmacy spirit (Figure 11-6). This simple but significant gesture may have a long-lasting impact on students' professional growth and development. May the pharmacy spirit be with you!

Figure 11-6 • Pharmacy Spirit Award

Pharmacy spirit is the energy, loyalty, dedication, and courage that pushes forward the frontiers of pharmacy practice. Pharmacy spirit is the heart and driving force behind providing and improving patient care. Pharmacy spirit is the enthusiasm, determination, and commitment, as well as the love, compassion, and kindness required for providing the best possible patient care. Pharmacy spirit is the soul of the pharmacy profession. Having pharmacy spirit symbolizes the ultimate commitment to the Pharmacy Oath, and therefore to the profession of pharmacy and to the public.

This distinguished Pharmacy Spirit Award is presented to ___________

on the __th day of ______ in the year ____.

Like a lighthouse ever shining light into the night to guide ships safely along their journey, you act as a beacon for the pharmacy profession by expressing pharmacy spirit and by leading pharmacists in the advancement of the practice of pharmacy and the care of patients.

____

Preceptor's Name

Preceptor's Title

Preceptor's Practice Site

References

1. Purcell K. Pharmacy spirit. Catch it! Newsletter. *Texas Society of Health-System Pharmacists.* 1995;24(9):3,6.
2. Description of pharmacy spirit. Available at: http://www.tshp.org/About/Organizational Documents.asp. Accessed March 1, 2005.

Appendix

Educational Outcomes

1. **Pharmaceutical Care**—Provide pharmaceutical care in cooperation with patients, prescribers, and other members of an interprofessional health care team based on sound therapeutic principles and evidence-based data, taking into account relevant legal, ethical, social, economic and professional issues, emerging technologies, and evolving biomedical, sociobehavioral, and clinical sciences that may impact therapeutic outcomes.
   a. Provide patient-centered care
      i. Design, implement, monitor, evaluate, and adjust pharmaceutical care plans that are patient-specific and evidence-based.
      ii. Communicate and collaborate with prescribers, patients, caregivers, and other involved health care providers to engender a team approach to patient care.
      iii. Retrieve, analyze, and interpret the professional, lay, and scientific literature to provide drug information to patients, their families, and other involved health care providers.
      iv. Carry out duties in accordance with legal, ethical, social economic, and professional guidelines.
      v. Maintain professional competence by identifying and analyzing emerging issues, products, and services that may impact patient-specific therapeutic outcomes.
   b. Provide population-based care
      i. Develop and implement population-specific, evidence-based disease management programs and protocols based on analysis of epidemiologic and pharmacoeconomic data, medication use criteria, medication use review, and risk reduction strategies.
      ii. Communicate and collaborate with prescribers, population members, caregivers, and other involved health care providers to engender a team approach to patient care.
      iii. Retrieve, analyze, and interpret the professional, lay, and scientific literature to provide drug information to patients, their families, and other involved health care providers.
      iv. Carry out duties in accordance with legal, ethical, social economic, and professional guidelines.

v. Maintain professional competence by identifying and analyzing emerging issues, products, and services that may impact patient-specific therapeutic outcomes.

2. **Systems Management**—Manage and use resources of the health care system, in cooperation with patients, prescribers, and other health care providers and administrative and supportive personnel, to promote health; to provide, assess, and coordinate safe, accurate, and time-sensitive medication distribution; and to improve therapeutic outcomes of medication use.

   a. Manage human, physical, medical, informational, and technological resources

      i. Apply relevant legal, ethical, social, economic, and professional principles/issues to assure efficient, cost-effective utilization of human, physical, medical, informational, and technological resources in the provision of patient care.

      ii. Communicate and collaborate with patients, prescribers, and other health care providers, and administrative and supportive personnel to engender a team approach to assure efficient, cost-effective utilization of human, physical, medical, informational, and technological resources in the provision of patient care.

      iii. Carry out duties in accordance with legal, ethical, social, economic, and professional guidelines.

      iv. Maintain professional competence by identifying and analyzing emerging issues, products, and services that may impact management of human, physical, medical, informational, and technological resources in the provision of patient care.

   b. Manage medication use systems

      i. Apply patient- and population-specific data, quality assurance strategies, and research processes to assure that medication use systems minimize drug misadventuring and optimize patient outcomes.

      ii. Apply patient- and population-specific data, quality assurance strategies, and research processes to develop drug use and health policy, and to design pharmacy benefits.

iii. Communicate and collaborate with prescribers, patients, caregivers, other involved health care providers and administrative and supportive personnel to identify and resolve medication use problems.

iv. Carry out duties in accordance with legal, ethical, social, economic, and professional guidelines.

v. Maintain professional competence by identifying and analyzing emerging issues, products, and services that may impact medication use systems, to develop use and health policy, and to design pharmacy benefits.

3. Public Health—Promote health improvement, wellness, and disease prevention in cooperation with patients, communities, at-risk populations, and other members of an interprofessional team of health care providers.

a. Assure the availability of effective, quality health and disease prevention services

i. Apply population-specific data, quality assurance strategies, and research processes to develop, identify and resolve public health problems.

ii. Communicate and collaborate with prescribers, policy makers, members of the community and other involved health care providers and administrative and supportive personnel to identify and resolve public health problems.

iii. Carry out duties in accordance with legal, ethical, social, economic, and professional guidelines.

iv. Maintain professional competence by identifying and analyzing emerging issues, products, and services that may affect the efficacy or quality of disease prevention services to amend existing or develop additional services.

b. Develop public health policy

i. Apply population-specific data, quality assurance strategies, and research processes to develop public health policy.

ii. Communicate and collaborate with prescribers, policy makers, members of the community, and other involved health care providers and administrative and supportive personnel to develop public policy.
iii. Carry out duties in accordance with legal, ethical, social economic, and professional guidelines.
iv. Maintain professional competence—by identifying and analyzing emerging issues, products, and services that may affect public health policy—to amend existing or develop additional policies.

Developed and revised by the American Association of Colleges of Pharmacy Center for the Advancement of Pharmaceutical Education (CAPE) Advisory Panel on Educational Outcomes, 2004.

Index

A

B

C

X–Z